NUTRITION
FOR
ADHD KIDS

ADJUSTING YOUR CHILD'S DIET TO ENHANCE FOCUS, SELF-REGULATE, AND DECREASE HYPERACTIVITY

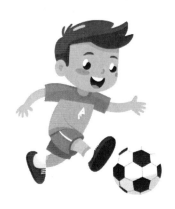

Maya Blackwood

© **Copyright 2024 - All rights reserved.**

The content contained within this book may not be reproduced, duplicated, or transmitted without direct written permission from the author or the publisher.

Under no circumstances will any blame or legal responsibility be held against the publisher or author for any damages, reparation, or monetary loss due to the information contained within this book, either directly or indirectly.

Legal Notice:

This book is copyright-protected. It is only for personal use. You cannot amend, distribute, sell, use, quote, or paraphrase any part or the content within this book without the consent of the author or publisher.

Disclaimer Notice:

Please note the information contained within this document is for educational and entertainment purposes only. All efforts have been executed to present accurate, up-to-date, reliable, and complete information. No warranties of any kind are declared or implied. Readers acknowledge that the author is not engaged in the rendering of legal, financial, medical, or professional advice. The content within this book has been derived from various sources. Please consult a licensed professional before attempting any techniques outlined in this book.

By reading this document, the reader agrees that under no circumstances is the author responsible for any losses, direct or indirect, that are incurred as a result of the use of the information contained within this document, including, but not limited to, errors, omissions, or inaccuracies.

Contents

Introduction   1
   Attention Deficit Hyperactivity Disorder and Nutrition
   What to Expect From This Book
   The Example of the Thompson Family

1. The Link Between Diet and ADHD Symptoms   7
      Exploring the Impact of Nutrition on ADHD Symptoms
      Omega-3 Fatty Acids
      Vitamins and Minerals
      Balanced Diet
      Food Additives and Sugar
      Identifying Common Dietary Triggers for Hyperactivity and Inattention
      Choosing to Embrace a Balanced Diet
      Jake's Breakthrough: Unveiling the Connection Between Diet and ADHD Symptom Management

2. Building a Healthy Foundation: The Basics of a Balanced Diet   21
      The Importance of Macronutrients and Micronutrients

Designing a Well-Rounded Meal Plan for Optimal Brain Health

Incorporating Whole Foods and Eliminating Processed Foods

Understanding How Nutrition Impacts ADHD Symptoms in Children

Jake's Nutritional Odyssey: Building a Strong Foundation With a Balanced Diet

3. Superfoods for ADHD Kids   37

Superfoods

The Power of Nutrient-Dense Foods in Supporting Cognitive Function for Children With ADHD

Key Nutrients for ADHD Management

Food and Ingredient Substitutions

What Healthy Snacks Are Suitable for Children With ADHD to Include in Their Diet?

Jake's Journey: Harnessing the Power of Superfoods to Manage ADHD Symptoms

4. Reducing Sugar and Artificial Additives   53

What Sugar and Artificial Additives Do to a Child With ADHD

Understanding the Effects of Sugar on Children With ADHD

Promoting Awareness and Determination

Learning to Read Food Labels and Identify Hidden Sugars

Foods to Steer Clear of if Your Child Has ADHD

Implementing Strategies for Reducing Sugar Cravings in Children

Sugar and ADHD in Kids: What's the Connection?

Sugar-Free Success: Jake's Journey to Healthier Eating Transforms His Family Dynamics

5. The Gut-Brain Connection: Healing the Gut for Improved Attention   67

    Discovering the Gut Microbiome

    Unlocking the Gut-Brain Connection: How Tummy Health Shapes ADHD Symptoms in Kids

    Exploring the Connection Between Gut Health and ADHD Symptoms

    Unraveling Food Sensitivities and ADHD: A Comprehensive Guide

    Unlocking the Power of Nutrition: Implementing an Elimination Diet for Managing ADHD Symptoms

    Implementing Gut-Healing Protocols and Incorporating Prebiotics for Digestive Health

    Tips for Nurturing a Healthy Gut in Children

    Gut Feeling: Jake's Journey to Improved Attention Through Healing His Gut-Brain Connection

6. Creating a Positive Mealtime Environment   83

    Strategies for Fostering Healthy Eating Habits and Positive Behaviors During Meals

    Encouraging Mindful Eating and Avoiding Distractions

    Involving Children in Meal Planning and Preparation to Increase Their Engagement

    Cooking Together: Age-Appropriate Kitchen Activities for Kids of All Ages

    Dealing With Selective Eaters at Mealtimes

    Streamlining the Eating Process for Picky Eaters

Feeding the Soul: Jake's Journey to Enjoying a Nurturing Mealtime Environment

7. Supplements and Alternative Therapies for ADHD Symptoms   101

Understanding the Role of Supplements in Supporting ADHD Symptoms

Exploring Holistic and Alternative Therapies to Complement Nutritional Interventions

Consulting With Health Care Professionals

Embracing a Holistic Approach to Managing Your Child's ADHD Symptoms

Jake's Journey: Exploring Supplements and Therapies for Managing ADHD Symptoms

8. Navigating School and Social Situations   115

Tips for Promoting Proper Nutrition at School and During Social Events

Communicating With Teachers and School Administration

Understanding the Importance of Open Communication

Jake's Triumph: Navigating School and Social Settings With ADHD

9. Lifestyle Factors for Optimal Brain Health   131

The Importance of Regular Exercise, Adequate Sleep, and Stress Reduction

Strategies for Incorporating Physical Activity Into Daily Routines

Exploring Relaxation Techniques and Mindfulness Practices for ADHD Kids

    Elevating Brain Health: Jake's Journey Through Lifestyle Optimization

Conclusion   147

    Parenting Tips for ADHD: Do's and Don'ts

    Taking a Holistic Approach

    A Message of Hope and Confidence

    Jake's ADHD Journey: A Tale of Resilience, Growth, and Advocacy

References   157

INTRODUCTION

Attention Deficit Hyperactivity Disorder and Nutrition

Attention deficit hyperactivity disorder (ADHD) is a neurological disorder that affects a significant number of children in the world. Over 6 million children in the United States alone grapple with it (Wirth, 2023). This is more than a statistic; it is a testament to the challenges faced by families daily.

At the core of the disorder lies a breakdown in communication between the prefrontal cortex, which can be visualized as a teacher in a bustling classroom, orchestrating attention and dampening distractions and other brain regions. When a child needs to concentrate but faces urges like an itch or restlessness, the prefrontal cortex guides them to focus on the most urgent task. However, when someone has ADHD, this essential communication system falters, resulting in a cacophony of background noise in the brain.

Symptoms of this disorder are categorized into inattention and hyperactivity-impulsivity. Inattention includes difficulty sustaining focus, careless mistakes, forgetfulness, and easy distractibility. Hyperactivity-impulsivity involves fidgeting, restlessness, impulsive decision-making, and difficulty waiting turns.

Those affected often struggle with these symptoms, as you may know from your experience, which can negatively impact academic performance, social interactions, and behavior. Because of this, challenges for children with ADHD span academics and social interactions: Focus issues in the classroom lead to academic struggles, while impulsive behavior and emotional immaturity can impact peer relationships.

Families face challenges in understanding and managing their child's behavior, necessitating collaboration with healthcare professionals, educators, and additional support networks to develop effective coping strategies. To successfully help children manage the disorder, it is essential to realize that personalized approaches are crucial. Each individual with ADHD is unique, and tailored treatment and support are ultimately what significantly contribute to thriving children.

While medication is a common treatment for ADHD, studies have shown that nutrition plays a critical role in managing symptoms (Lange et al., 2023). Numerous studies suggest that nutrition can influence a child's focus, self-regulation, and hyperactivity. Diet alone may not be the sole cause of ADHD, but there is evidence supporting the idea that certain dietary factors can affect symptoms.

By reassessing your child's meal plan and making healthier food choices, you can provide them with the necessary nutrients to improve their symptoms and promote their overall health and well-being. A well-balanced diet that includes whole grains, fruits, vegetables, proteins, and healthy fats can help improve focus, reduce hyperactivity, and enhance cognitive function.

What to Expect From This Book

Welcome to the transformative world of *Nutrition for ADHD Kids*, where every meal can potentially change the lives of children with ADHD.

In a society filled with alternative treatments, some effective and others not, people often search for solutions beyond conventional approaches. It is remarkable that in a world brimming with distractions, assisting your child in finding focus and tranquility might be as straightforward as re-evaluating their meal plan.

Until you stumbled upon this book, did you ever ponder whether altering their diet could impact their ADHD symptoms? The contents of these chapters will show you that the key to unlocking your child's potential lies not just in textbooks and therapy but also in the carefully curated choices on their dinner plate.

In this book, you will explore the intricate connection between nutrition and ADHD symptoms, which scientific insights and real-life experiences have backed. Armed with facts and curiosity, you'll embark on this journey and unravel the story of nutrition's profound influence on ADHD symptoms. You will also explore how specific nutrients catalyze improved focus, enhanced self-regulation, and overall well-being.

However, this book isn't just about meals but about empowering parents with practical strategies, expert insights, and a comprehensive toolkit to navigate the dynamic relationship between nutrition and ADHD. So, as you delve into the chapters, you will decode problem foods, learn how to build a balanced diet, explore the role of supplements, and find insights on how to create a supportive environment for your child.

The Example of the Thompson Family

The Thompson family, known for their spirited child, resided in a tranquil neighborhood with their energetic son. From an early age, the boy's zest for life hinted at a unique quality that could be tied to his ADHD diagnosis.

Meet Jake, a remarkable individual whose journey with ADHD is a testament to resilience, growth, and the power of self-discovery. From his early days navigating the challenges of school to his ongoing quest for understanding and acceptance, Jake's path with ADHD is both enlightening and inspiring.

Through navigating life's ups and downs, the Thompsons discovered their journey would be as unique as the fingerprints on Jake's hands. His first day of school remains a standout memory. With his brimming excitement, his boundless energy clashed with the traditional classroom, initiating a daily struggle to sit still and focus that would follow him for years.

The real challenge, however, extended beyond school. The Thompsons eventually realized that Jake's behavior was linked to his nutrition and that the remedy wasn't just about avoiding sugary treats. As a family, they navigated the challenge of comprehending the connection between Jake's diet and his struggle with impulse regulation.

As they tried one strategy after another, navigating Jake's meal preparations became akin to embarking on a thrilling adventure. For a while, mornings were a battlefield. Each day presented the challenge of concocting a breakfast that provided sustenance without inciting hyperactivity, turning it into a test of patience and precision for the Thompsons.

At lunchtime, Jake's aversion to certain tastes was a determined challenge. His parents managed the obstacle by ingeniously incorporating nutrient-dense foods into their son's favorite lunchbox items. Playing with color and finding stealthy ways to include plenty of vegetables, they turned midday meals into playful presentations that sparked Jake's imagination.

When it came to the social domain, the Thompsons confronted their initial frustrations with fortitude. They became adept at preparing alternative but delicious treats for birthday parties and playdates, maintaining a balance that supported Jake's well-being.

As they faced these challenges, the family found a supportive community of parents, who, through the exchange of tips and emotional support, turned Jake's journey into a collective resilience effort. This community, including Jake's teachers, witnessed remarkable progress in the following years. Careful attention to nutrition and strategies for channeling positive energy shifted overwhelming hurdles into stepping stones for Jake's self-discovery and success.

The Thompson family's story illuminates the multifaceted nature of raising a child with ADHD—it shows that it is not just managing behavior but also understanding the intricate interplay between nutrition, environment, and individual strengths. In recognizing Jake's unique brilliance, the family could find new ways to celebrate his vibrant, resilient, and endlessly curious personality.

The great news is that you, too, can discover the game-changing power of nutrition. It can transform your child's life and pave the way for enhanced focus, improved behavior, and a brighter future. The time has now come for you to challenge and question the conventional wisdom related to the treatment of ADHD and introduce nutrition as an alternative or complementary approach that can significantly impact your child's well-being.

This book will continue this introspective journey into the Thompson family's example. We'll delve into Jake's experiences, exploring the highs and lows, triumphs and setbacks, and valuable lessons he has learned. Through his story, we'll uncover the complexities of ADHD, its impact on daily life, and the strategies to manage its symptoms effectively.

Join us as we follow Jake on his quest for self-understanding, empowerment, and, ultimately, a sense of belonging in a world where ADHD is not a limitation but rather an aspect of his unique identity.

THE LINK BETWEEN DIET AND ADHD SYMPTOMS

Let's take the first steps to manage attention deficit hyperactivity disorder (ADHD). We will unravel the incredible impact of diet on ADHD symptoms. Prepare to navigate through a mosaic of daily choices, where each morsel and sip contributes to the intricate tapestry of life, potentially paving the way for improved well-being and clarity for you and your child.

This chapter dissects the science behind the dietary connection, unraveling the biological intricacies that tie nutrition to brain functioning. Through compelling research, we will highlight the tangible impact of food choices on ADHD symptoms—these range from the overt manifestations of hyperactivity to the subtler shades of inattention. The dietary connection emerges as a powerful lever influencing the fabric of your child's cognitive experience.

We will zoom in on the pivotal role of nutrition in managing ADHD symptoms, backed not just by hypotheses but by compelling evidence from a burgeoning field of study. We'll delve into the labyrinth of nutrients and dietary triggers to understand their intricate dance with the manifestations of this attention disorder. Certain nutrients will emerge as protagonists, capable of alleviating challenges, while we'll see that others act as antagonists, exacerbating complex symptoms.

We'll explore dietary strategies to manage ADHD symptoms with insights and expert advice, empowering you to make informed decisions about your child's nutrition. As we delve deeper into the relationship between diet and ADHD, you'll learn that every food and drink choice holds the potential to contribute to a brighter, more focused tomorrow.

Exploring the Impact of Nutrition on ADHD Symptoms

The intersection of nutrition, impulsivity, and hyperactivity symptoms is a nuanced and multifaceted subject, continuously evolving as researchers delve deeper into the relationship between the two. As we commence this exploration, let's unravel some key insights regarding the potential impact of nutrition on ADHD symptoms.

It is essential to recognize that while certain dietary patterns may exacerbate symptoms, others hold promise in mitigating their severity. For example, diets rich in omega-3 fatty acids, antioxidants, and essential vitamins and minerals have shown potential for alleviation. Conversely, diets high in refined sugars, artificial additives, and processed foods may exacerbate inattention and excessive, unrestrained movement.

Consider individual variability, as each child's response to dietary interventions may differ. Genetic predisposition, metabolic differences, and environmental factors can influence how the body and brain respond to nutritional changes.

Additionally, the gut-brain connection has emerged as a fascinating area of study, with growing evidence suggesting that digestive health may play an essential role in modulating symptoms. Research indicates that imbalances in gut microbiota, inflammation, and intestinal permeability may contribute to neurodevelopmental disorders like ADHD (Iliodromiti et al., 2023). Thus, interventions aimed at optimizing gut health through dietary modifications, probiotics, and prebiotics hold promise in managing the condition.

Nutritional interventions impact more than symptom management: They influence cognitive function, emotional regulation, and overall well-being. By prioritizing nutrient-dense foods and avoiding potential dietary triggers, parents such as yourself can create an environment conducive to your child's optimal development.

So, you can see how the relationship between nutrition and ADHD symptoms is complex and shaped by dietary factors, individual differences, and physiological mechanisms. Understanding these nuances and implementing evidence-based dietary strategies empowers you to support your child's holistic health amid challenges.

Omega-3 Fatty Acids

Brain Development

Omega-3 fatty acids, found in fatty fish like salmon, play a crucial role in the intricate blueprint of children's brain development. These essential fat building blocks are not merely passive spectators; they actively shape the foundation of neural architecture. Specifically, omega-3s contribute to constructing cell membranes, the protective sheaths that envelop and nourish brain cells.

These nutritional components are akin to the developers of a burgeoning metropolis. They ensure the stability and flexibility of the structural framework supporting the cacophony of activity. In brain development, omega-3s act as indispensable builders, laying the groundwork for robust neuron communication and signaling pathways.

Cognitive Benefits

Optimal levels of omega-3 fatty acids, especially EPA and DHA, have cognitive advantages. These unsung heroes of the dietary world may hold the key to enhancing mental prowess, especially for children grappling with ADHD.

Picture EPA and DHA as conductors orchestrating a concerto within your child's brain. Research suggests that these specific omega-3s harmonize neuronal activities, influencing attention and refining the symphony of focus (Pearson, 2017). Because of this function, they may contribute to a cognitive landscape where attention and focus can flourish by fostering an environment conducive to efficient neurotransmission.

In the elaborate tapestry of your child's cognitive development, omega-3 fatty acids emerge as building blocks and active agents that sculpt a landscape where neurons communicate with finesse. As you explore the intersection of nutrition and cognitive function, the role of these fatty acids becomes increasingly apparent: They perform a nuanced dance of brain development, and cognitive enhancement unfolds with each nutrient-rich bite.

Vitamins and Minerals

Iron and Dopamine Production

Iron conducts attention and motivation in the intricate symphony of neurotransmitters that oversee your child's cognitive functions. This vital mineral is pivotal in producing dopamine, a chemical in the brain celebrated for influencing focus and drive. You can imagine iron as the catalyst, orchestrating the synthesis of dopamine to create a harmonious rhythm within your child's brain.

Ensuring that kids receive an ample supply of iron through dietary sources like lean meats and beans is more than a nutritional consideration when ADHD is involved—it becomes a fundamental investment in their cognitive health. Iron-rich foods can be compared to maestros guiding the creation of a neurotransmitter composition that propels your child's attention and motivation to new heights.

Zinc and Neurotransmitter Regulation

Zinc is a skilled regulator in the neural network that forms the foundation of the human cognitive landscape. It fine-tunes the delicate dance of neural signaling molecules, including the pivotal dopamine, which you've just learned about. This vital mineral assumes the role of a choreographer, ensuring that the neurotransmitter performances unfold with precision and grace.

Adequate levels of zinc are like a backstage director, contributing to optimal neuronal communication and supporting the orchestration of a symphony of attention and focus in your child. Envision zinc-rich foods as the prima ballerinas in this regulatory ensemble, guiding the neurotransmitter interactions with finesse. By maintaining a delicate balance, the mineral supports the nuanced dance of neurotransmitters, creating an environment where attention and focus can take center stage.

Iron and zinc emerge as indispensable components in the nutritional narrative of your child's cognitive well-being, each playing a role in shaping the symphony of neurotransmitters. By making dietary choices rich in these essential minerals, you nurture their bodies and actively contribute to the intricate biochemical ballet that defines their cognitive health.

Balanced Diet

Nutrient-Rich Foods

On the culinary journey to nourishing the body and the intricate workings of your child's mind, a well-balanced diet is a potent elixir for intellectual well-being. Imagine it as a canvas painted with a rich array of nutrients, each contributing its unique essence to the masterpiece of neurotransmitter function. This nutritional composition, comprised of vibrant fruits, verdant vegetables, nourishing whole grains, fortifying lean proteins, and the harmonious hum of healthy fats, is the bedrock from which cognitive brilliance takes shape.

In this gastronomic kaleidoscope, fruits offer the sweetness of antioxidants, vegetables unveil a palette of vitamins and minerals, whole grains provide sustained energy, lean proteins supply essential amino acids, and healthy fats add nuanced richness. The amalgamation of these elements goes beyond mere sustenance—it becomes a dance routine choreographed to support the rhythm of neurotransmitters and orchestrate a harmonious interplay for your child's overall cognitive performance.

Protein and Neurotransmitter Production

Zooming into the microscopic ballet within your child's neural landscape, proteins emerge as virtuosos, playing a transformative role in the production of neurotransmitters. Whether sourced from the juiciness of meats or the wholesomeness of legumes, proteins shape mood regulation and attention pathways. They act as alchemists, transmuting into the essential building blocks for neurotransmitters like serotonin, dopamine, and norepinephrine.

Picture each protein-rich bite of your child's meals as a note in the chorus of cognitive wellness, contributing to the vibrant notes of mood stability and focused attention. The amino acids derived from these sources become the threads weaving through the intricate fabric of your child's neurological development, enhancing physical vitality and the essence of mental well-being.

As you curate a diet rich in diverse nutrients and protein sources, you are crafting meals and sculpting the foundation of your child's mental vitality. This nutritional masterpiece, painted with the brushstrokes of wholesome variety and the precision of protein's influence, nurtures the flourishing landscape of neurotransmitters and supports the symphony of cognitive brilliance in your child's life.

Food Additives and Sugar

Additives and Hyperactivity

We can now venture into dietary considerations, noting that some studies have delved into the potential influence of specific food additives on hyperactivity, particularly in children. While the evidence remains a subject of ongoing exploration, researchers acknowledge that certain individuals may exhibit sensitivity to these synthetic ingredients.

Additives are subtle notes in the dietary composition, potentially influencing the tempo of hyperactivity in some children. In their scientific exploration, researchers operate as musical critics, meticulously examining the dietary landscape to understand how these notes might contribute to variations in behavior. In their consideration of the evidence, the score of individual responses unfolds with nuance. We see that what may be inconsequential for some could resonate differently in the behavior of others. As we navigate this intriguing intersection of diet and hyperactivity, recognizing the potential impact of additives becomes a step toward crafting dietary strategies tailored to individual sensitivities.

Sugar Moderation

The debate surrounding the relationship between sugar and ADHD continues to echo through nutritional discussions. Sugar is a double-edged sword—it provides momentary sweetness but potentially contributes to fluctuations in blood sugar levels. While a definitive link remains elusive, moderation has emerged as a prudent approach for holistically improving your child's symptoms.

Moderation is a compass guiding the way to meals that mitigate the peaks and valleys of spiked blood sugar. Balanced meals are stabilizers, helping your child maintain a steady current of energy that influences their physical health and attention span. They sustain your child's focus and cognitive equilibrium.

In the ongoing discourse between science and dietary choices, the potential impact of additives and the nuanced relationship with sugar moderation paint a portrait of considerations for parents and caregivers. Each child's nutritional journey is a unique artwork shaped by evidence and the subtleties of personal response. Navigating these dietary considerations requires a balance of scientific awareness and individualized approaches.

Unique Responses

Understanding the impact of nutrition on ADHD symptoms unveils a profound truth—each child's response to nutritional interventions is as distinctive as their fingerprint. There is a spectrum of individual reactions, and what proves to be an elixir for one child may not necessarily be the magic potion for another. The dynamics of each child's physiology, metabolism, and nutritional needs form a unique network that influences how they respond to dietary changes.

This uniqueness is a kaleidoscope of varied sensitivities, preferences, and genetic predispositions. It shapes the landscape of dietary impact with subtle intricacies. As caregivers, parents, and educators navigate the path of nutritional choices, recognizing these individual responses guides personalized approaches. Understanding that there is no one-size-fits-all solution but rather a range of nuanced individualities invites a tailored and empathetic approach to support children with ADHD through nutrition.

Professional Guidance

When grappling with nutrition and neurodevelopment, seeking professional guidance emerges as a beacon of wisdom. Pediatricians and registered dietitians are expert navigators who will chart a course based on your child's unique needs and health status. Envision them as skilled cartographers, mapping out a personalized nutritional journey that considers not only the symptoms of inattention, impulsivity, and hyperactivity but also your child's holistic well-being.

As you embark on this collaborative journey with health professionals, a wealth of personalized insights will unfold. These experts can become partners in decoding the complex language of your child's nutritional needs, offering tailored recommendations that exceed generic advice. They provide a road map through consultations where dietary considerations align with your child's medical history, sensitivities, and developmental milestones. This collaborative approach will ensure that the nutritional strategies implemented are evidence-based and finely tuned to your child's health and lifestyle.

As a parent, you can find harmonious notes that resonate with your child's well-being in the symphony of unique responses and professional guidance. Exploring this complex domain becomes a shared endeavor, and individualized care and expert insights converge to create a nuanced and impactful approach to nutrition and ADHD management.

As you nourish your child's well-being, these critical insights guide you through the personalized landscape of nutrition and its potential impact on ADHD symptoms. It's not just about theories and scientific principles; it's about your child, their needs, and the rhythms of your family life.

In weaving together the threads of scientific knowledge and individualized guidance, your aim should be to understand and actively participate in crafting strategies to enhance your child's journey. This isn't a singular approach; it's a tailored expedition that accounts for your child's responses and preferences.

In this collaborative endeavor, your insights as a parent meld seamlessly with the expertise of healthcare professionals. Together, you become architects of a holistic approach that considers not just the impact on ADHD symptoms but the entirety of your child's wellness—their joys, challenges, and the daily motions that make your family unique.

The goal of working with a knowledgeable team is clear: to unlock strategies that go beyond theory and become living, breathing practices that enhance your child's well-being. Through this personalized approach, you're not just following a predetermined route; you're actively shaping a path that aligns with your family's heartbeat and contributes to your child's vibrant health and happiness.

Identifying Common Dietary Triggers for Hyperactivity and Inattention

While your child is unique and individual responses to foods vary, certain dietary elements have been widely acknowledged as potential exacerbating factors for ADHD symptoms. Because it is pivotal for crafting effective management plans, you must be able to both recognize and understand common food triggers that can worsen hyperactivity and inattention in children with ADHD.

Let's delve deeper into some of these prominent culprits:

Artificial Food Additives

Many artificial additives, such as synthetic colors like tartrazine and sunset yellow FCF, preservatives like sodium benzoate, and flavor enhancers like monosodium glutamate, have been associated with heightened hyperactivity and decreased attention in children with ADHD. These additives are prevalent in processed foods, sugary beverages, candies, and snacks, making them essential to avoid.

Sugar and Refined Carbohydrates

Although sugar itself doesn't directly cause ADHD, consuming too many high-sugar drinks and foods can lead to rapid fluctuations in blood sugar levels, which may worsen symptoms. This roller-coaster effect can result in energy crashes and difficulties in maintaining focus and attention. Similarly, foods rich in refined carbohydrates, like white bread, pasta, and pastries, can induce sharp spikes in blood sugar levels, followed by behavioral disturbances.

Highly Processed Foods

Processed foods often contain high levels of sugar, unhealthy fats, and artificial additives, which can adversely affect brain function and exacerbate ADHD symptoms. These foods include fast food, frozen meals, sugary cereals, and packaged snacks, making them important targets to minimize in your child's diet.

Allergens and Sensitivities

Some children with ADHD may exhibit sensitivities or allergies to certain foods like dairy, gluten, soy, eggs, or nuts. Consuming them can trigger inflammatory responses and immune reactions, potentially worsening their inattention and hyperactivity. Identifying and eliminating these trigger foods can be crucial for symptom management.

Caffeine and High-Energy Drinks

Caffeine, a stimulant found in coffee, tea, energy drinks, and some sodas, can exacerbate agitation and impulsivity in children with ADHD.

High-energy drinks, often laden with caffeine and sugar, can further intensify hyperactivity and inattention, making it advisable to limit or avoid these beverages.

Omega-6 Fatty Acids

Despite omega-3's potential benefits for brain health, consuming an unbalanced ratio of omega-3 and omega-6 fatty acids may worsen ADHD symptoms by causing inflammation. Foods high in omega-6 fatty acids, like corn and soybean oil, and processed snacks should be avoided.

Choosing to Embrace a Balanced Diet

When you, as a parent, can identify and minimize your child's exposure to these common dietary triggers, you can play a crucial role in alleviating their symptoms and enhancing their overall health. Shifting to a balanced diet rich in whole foods provides essential nutrients for optimal brain function and may mitigate the impact of dietary factors on ADHD symptoms. Additionally, seeking guidance from your family doctor or a registered dietitian can offer an avenue to personalized strategies for managing your child's nutritional triggers.

In the next chapter, you'll discover ways to support your child with ADHD's health. You will explore how nutrition can play an important role in managing their symptoms and learn about the basics of a balanced diet tailored specifically for children with the disorder. You will receive practical advice and valuable insights to enhance your child's well-being.

Additionally, you will learn about essential nutrition principles and practical tips to support your child's growth and development. We'll discuss the importance of incorporating nutrient-rich foods and strategies to minimize potential triggers that could worsen your child's ADHD symptoms.

Jake's Breakthrough: Unveiling the Connection Between Diet and ADHD Symptom Management

Jake's exploration of nutrition as a means to manage his ADHD symptoms, starting in his childhood with his parents' support and continuing as he has matured, is truly inspiring. Let us delve into its positive impact on various aspects of his life.

Jake's experience with managing his ADHD symptoms through a balanced diet is a testament to how dietary changes can have a positive impact on overall wellness. By incorporating nutrient-rich foods such as fish and leafy greens into Jake's meals when he was still a child, Jake's parents witnessed him experience a significant reduction in hyperactivity and inattention. Maintaining this dietary habit as he matured has led to his cognitive function improving, focus sharpening, and memory boosting over the long term.

By being mindful of his parents' guidance on the impact that food additives and refined sugars can have on his ADHD symptoms, Jake has been able to cut back on processed foods. This has allowed him to reduce his intake of unhealthy treats, leading to more stable focus and attention throughout the day. By carefully monitoring his diet and paying attention to how different foods affect him, he has empowered himself to make informed choices that support his overall well-being.

Therefore, Jake's journey reminds us of the profound impact nutrition can have on managing ADHD and overall brain health. By prioritizing a balanced diet, we can all fuel our brains with the nutrients they need to function at their best and improve our quality of life.

BUILDING A HEALTHY FOUNDATION: THE BASICS OF A BALANCED DIET

Nutrition is a cornerstone for well-being in the sophisticated circuitry of childhood development, where growth, development, and exploration intertwine. For children trying to overcome the challenges of ADHD, a balanced diet is even more pivotal, as it offers a sturdy foundation for physical vitality and cognitive resilience.

In this chapter, you will explore the fundamental principles of a nutrition plan tailored specifically for children with ADHD. Let's dive into the essentials of a balanced diet and discover how it shapes attention, focus, and behavior. Together, we will unlock the keys to nourishing the body and the mind for a vibrant future.

As you forage further into the world of nutrition, you will uncover the core components of a balanced diet, from macronutrients to micronutrients and their well-choreographed dance within the body and mind. You will see the path toward nourishing the body and brain for optimal performance illuminated through practical insights and actionable strategies.

Join us as we lay the groundwork of a healthy foundation, approaching each meal as an opportunity to fuel growth, support cognitive function, and foster resilience in children with ADHD. Let's set sail on a voyage toward holistic health and vibrant vitality for our children. Together, we can empower other parents and caregivers like you to become champions in their child's holistic well-being!

The Importance of Macronutrients and Micronutrients

Macronutrients, including carbohydrates, proteins, and fats, are the foundational pillars of your child's diet. They provide the energy and important building blocks for growth, development, and daily activities.

Carbohydrates are the primary energy source for both the brain and the body. They provide readily available fuel to support cognitive functions. Meanwhile, proteins play a vital role in tissue repair and neurotransmitter synthesis, contributing to improved focus and mood regulation. On the other hand, fats, particularly omega-3 fatty acids, are essential for brain development, nerve function, and overall cognitive health, influencing attention span and behavioral outcomes.

As a parent or caregiver, you can optimize your child's brain health and reduce ADHD symptoms by ensuring a diverse, nutrient-rich diet with sufficient micronutrients. These vitamins and minerals act as vital co-factors and antioxidants, facilitating various biochemical reactions and protecting the brain from oxidative stress. For example, the vitamin B complex is crucial in neurotransmitter synthesis, while minerals like iron and zinc support cognitive function and mood stability.

Additionally, mindful planning and preparation can help ensure that each meal is nutritionally balanced and meets your child's specific dietary needs. By prioritizing nutrient-dense foods and minimizing the consumption of processed and sugary snacks, you can provide the essential nutrients required for optimal brain function and behavioral regulation.

Designing a Well-Rounded Meal Plan for Optimal Brain Health

It is important to prioritize a wholesome meal plan for children with ADHD to support their brain health and management of their symptoms. A balanced diet of nutrient-dense whole foods provides essential nutrients for cognitive function and emotional regulation. Prioritizing options high in omega-3 fatty acids, complex carbohydrates, lean proteins, and healthy fats supports sustained energy levels and improves focus and attention.

Consistency in meal times and choices also reinforces healthy eating habits, offering stability in daily routines. By minimizing processed foods, including microwave meals, cakes and cookies, and savory snacks like potato chips, you can reduce inflammation and oxidative stress, which may exacerbate ADHD symptoms.

Ultimately, a well-rounded meal plan supports brain function and fosters physical health, empowering children with ADHD to thrive academically and emotionally. Here's a step-by-step guide to help you create such a meal plan:

- **Start with a balanced plate:** Aim for colorful options to ensure a diverse range of nutrients and encourage meals that incorporate a variety of food groups, including fruits, vegetables, whole grains, lean proteins, and healthy fats.

- **Include omega-3 fatty acids:** Omega-3s are essential for brain health and can help improve attention and focus. Incorporate foods rich in omega-3 fatty acids, like fatty fish such as mackerel and sardines, flaxseeds, chia seeds, and walnuts.

- **Prioritize protein:** Protein-rich foods provide the amino acids necessary for neurotransmitter production, which can help regulate mood and behavior. Include lean meats, poultry, eggs, tofu, legumes, and nuts.

- **Opt for complex carbohydrates:** Choose complex carbohydrates over simple sugars to maintain steady energy levels. Some options include whole grains like oats, quinoa, brown rice, and whole-grain bread.

- **Add a variety of vegetables**: Including vegetables in your family's meals is a great idea. Combining them with protein and healthy fats will enhance your diet, and they can contribute to improved appetite regulation and digestive health.

- **Emphasize antioxidant-rich foods:** Antioxidants protect brain cells from damage and inflammation. To provide variety, include colorful fruits and vegetables like berries, spinach, kale, carrots, and bell peppers.

- **Mindful hydration:** Ensure your child stays hydrated throughout the day, as dehydration can affect cognitive function. Offer water as the primary beverage and limit sugary drinks.

- **Portion control:** Pay attention to your child's portion sizes to support weight management and prevent overeating. The plate method divides the plate into half for vegetables and the other half into quarters for protein and grains, which can guide portion sizes.

- **Snack smart:** Offer nutritious snacks between meals to keep energy levels stable. Opt for fruit with nut butter, yogurt with berries, or veggies with hummus.

- **Consistency is key:** Establish regular meal and snack times to promote orderly eating habits. Consistent nutrition can help stabilize mood and improve overall behavior.

- **Get children involved:** Encourage children to participate in meal planning and preparation. This can increase their interest in healthy foods and empower them to make nutritious choices.

By following these steps and incorporating various nutrient-rich foods into your family's daily meals, you can create a well-rounded meal plan that supports optimal brain health for a child with ADHD. Remember that even small changes over time can lead to significant improvements.

Incorporating Whole Foods and Eliminating Processed Foods

Incorporating whole foods and eliminating processed foods from an ADHD child's diet can have immense positive effects on their attention, behavior, and overall health. Whole foods, rich in essential nutrients like vitamins, minerals, and antioxidants, support optimal brain function and cognitive development.

By prioritizing nutrient-dense options like fruits, vegetables, whole grains, lean proteins, and healthy fats, you provide your child with the building blocks necessary for sustained energy, improved focus, and enhanced mood regulation. Conversely, processed foods that are high in refined sugars, unhealthy fats, and artificial additives can exacerbate their symptoms by causing energy spikes and crashes, mood swings, and difficulty concentrating.

Transitioning to a Diet Centered on Whole Foods

Transitioning to a diet centered around whole, unprocessed foods not only addresses nutritional needs but also reduces the intake of potentially harmful substances, promoting better overall health and well-being for children with ADHD.

Detrimental Effects of Processed Foods

The food industry purposefully adds high-fructose corn syrup and unhealthy fats into products to enhance their addictiveness. Research suggests that the blend of sugar, salt, and fat can affect the brain similarly to the way addictive drugs do (Schaefer & Yasin, 2020). Regularly consuming these foods can lead to health problems like obesity, heart disease, diabetes, and cancer. Therefore, eating nutrient-dense whole foods rather than processed ones is vital for overall family health.

Benefits of Whole Foods

Consuming nutrient-dense whole foods has numerous advantages, including stabilizing energy levels and supporting cognitive function. They also provide important vitamins, minerals, and antioxidants that help promote brain health and mitigate ADHD symptoms.

Practical Suggestions for Transitioning

Here are some practical suggestions for gradually transitioning toward a diet rich in nutritious foods. These tips consider the fact that taste buds change every two weeks and that repeated tastings over 2–4 weeks can help children learn to enjoy new foods. By following these condensed steps and being patient, you can transition your child toward a diet rich in nutritious foods while allowing their taste buds to adapt and evolve. Our accompanying workbook can help you keep track of the changes you're about to make.

Let us delve deeper into each section of our sample meal plan and transition guide.

Week 1

- **Breakfast:** Transitioning from sugary breakfasts to a less processed option is a significant first step. Choose cereals that are higher in fiber and lower in added sugars to provide sustained energy and improve focus throughout the morning. Encourage kids to explore new flavors and textures by adding fresh fruit or a sprinkle of cinnamon to their cereal.

- **Lunch:** A turkey and cheese sandwich on whole-grain bread offers a balanced combination of protein, carbohydrates, and healthy fats. Whole grain bread provides fiber for sustained energy, while turkey and cheese offer essential nutrients like protein and calcium. Pair the sandwich with crunchy carrot sticks and sweet apple slices for a satisfying midday meal.

- **Dinner:** Baked chicken tenders are a kid-friendly option that's easy to prepare and packed with protein. As accompaniments, sweet potatoes offer a rich source of vitamins and minerals, including vitamin A and potassium, while broccoli provides fiber and antioxidants. This balanced dinner ensures that kids receive the essential nutrients for their health.

Week 2

- **Breakfast:** Instant oatmeal is a convenient and nutritious option for busy mornings. Look for varieties that are lower in added sugars and that offer natural flavors like cinnamon or vanilla. Allow kids to personalize their oatmeal by adding toppings such as fresh fruit, nuts, or a drizzle of honey for added sweetness.

- **Lunch:** A pasta salad is a versatile dish that can be customized with various ingredients. When you make it, use whole-grain pasta for added fiber and nutrients. Bulk it up by incorporating colorful veggies like bell peppers, cherry tomatoes, and cucumbers for extra nutrition. Finish it with grilled chicken strips, which add protein to satisfy kids until their next meal.

- **Dinner:** Homemade pizza is a fun and interactive meal for the whole family. Use whole wheat crust for added fiber and nutrients, and complete it with tomato sauce, veggies, and lean proteins like chicken or turkey sausage. Let kids get creative with their toppings to make mealtime more enjoyable and engaging.

Week 3

- **Breakfast:** Rolled oats are a nutritious, filling breakfast option that provides sustained energy throughout the morning. Sweeten the porridge with a small amount of brown sugar or honey for added flavor, and encourage kids to add their favorite fruits or nuts for extra texture and nutritional value.

- **Lunch:** Quinoa salad is a nutrient-dense meal that's perfect for lunchtime. Quinoa is a complete protein and a good source of fiber, making it an ideal option for kids with ADHD. Combine it with fresh veggies like cucumber, tomatoes, and feta cheese for a refreshing and flavorful dish. Add grilled shrimp for added protein and a burst of flavor.

- **Dinner:** Baked salmon is a delicious dinner option rich in brain-healthy omega-3 fatty acids. Serve the fish with quinoa pilaf, a hearty grain option high in protein and fiber, and steamed green beans for added vitamins and minerals.

Week 4

- **Breakfast:** Sweeten rolled oats naturally with dates or maple syrup for a healthier alternative to refined sugars. Pureed dates add natural sweetness and a rich, caramel-like flavor to the oats, while maple syrup provides a deliciously sweet finish. Encourage kids to top their oats with nuts, seeds, or coconut flakes for added crunch and texture.

- **Lunch:** A veggie wrap is a colorful lunch option packed with fiber, vitamins, and minerals. To make it, spread hummus on a whole-grain wrap and fill it with shredded carrots, spinach, and sliced turkey or tofu.

- **Dinner:** Stir-fried tofu or chicken with mixed vegetables served over brown rice is a beautiful dinner option. As a method, stir-frying allows you to retain the nutrients and flavors of the ingredients while cooking them quickly over high heat. Brown rice offers fiber and complex carbohydrates to keep kids feeling full and energized.

This gradual four-week meal plan offers a structured approach to transitioning children with ADHD to healthier eating habits. By starting with familiar foods and gradually introducing nutrient-rich alternatives, you can support their overall well-being and cognitive function.

Remember to involve children in meal planning and preparation, celebrate their progress, and approach each week creatively and positively. With consistency and patience, you can empower your child with ADHD to embrace a diet that fuels their bodies and minds for success.

Tips for Grocery Shopping and Meal Preparation

- Choose fresh, seasonal produce and prioritize organic options when possible.

- Avoid the center aisles of the grocery store, where processed foods are typically located. Instead, focus on the perimeter, where whole foods like vegetables, fruits, meats, and dairy products are found.

- Cook and prepare meals in advance to save time and ensure nutritious meals are available throughout the week.

- Encouraging children to be involved in grocery shopping and meal preparation fosters a positive relationship with food and reinforces healthy eating habits.

This section has illuminated the harmful impacts of processed foods, underscored the advantages of whole foods, and offered actionable tips for transitioning to a healthier diet. It has empowered you to enact meaningful changes that bolster the vitality of children grappling with ADHD.

Understanding How Nutrition Impacts ADHD Symptoms in Children

Unraveling the intricate relationship between diet and neurodevelopmental disorders, particularly ADHD, involves understanding which foods can exacerbate symptoms. This is crucial for guiding you as a parent toward making informed dietary decisions.

Numerous studies have highlighted the significant impact of specific dietary components on cognitive function, mood regulation, and behavior, shedding light on the importance of nutrition in managing the condition. Empowering you with this knowledge has equipped you to make proactive choices that can positively influence your child's well-being and long-term health outcomes.

Moreover, highly processed foods, laden with unhealthy fats and devoid of essential nutrients, may exacerbate symptoms by promoting inflammation and oxidative stress, further compromising neurobehavioral function. To mitigate these effects, you must be vigilant and consider dietary modifications, prioritizing whole, nutrient-rich options. This includes eliminating potential allergens or sensitivities like gluten, dairy, and food dyes, which can trigger or worsen ADHD symptoms in some children.

Taking a proactive approach to nutrition empowers you to optimize your child's well-being. By embracing whole foods rich in essential vitamins, minerals, and antioxidants, you can lay the foundation for optimal brain health and development. Furthermore, incorporating omega-3 fatty acid-rich foods like tuna and anchovies, soybeans, and hemp seeds can support cognitive function and mitigate symptoms, including excessive movement, difficulty with turn-taking, and constant interruption.

Navigating this intricate terrain of nutrition and ADHD requires a comprehensive understanding of dietary influences and their implications. By adopting the balanced approach we have emphasized, you can chart a course toward improved cognitive function for your child. Through collaboration with healthcare professionals and dietitians, you can tailor dietary interventions to meet your child's unique needs and preferences, ultimately empowering them to thrive and reach their full potential.

Key Culprits

- **Artificial food additives:** Synthetic colorings, flavorings, and preservatives found in processed snacks and sodas have been linked to increased hyperactivity and impulsivity.

- **Refined sugars:** Sugary snacks and beverages can cause rapid fluctuations in blood sugar levels, contributing to energy crashes and worsening ADHD symptoms.

- **Highly processed foods:** Loaded with unhealthy fats and lacking essential nutrients may promote inflammation and oxidative stress, compromising neurobehavioral function.

- **Allergens or sensitivities:** Certain foods like gluten, dairy, and food dyes can trigger or worsen ADHD symptoms in susceptible children.

Practical Strategies

- **Balanced macronutrients:** Incorporate sufficient protein, healthy fats, and complex carbohydrates to stabilize blood sugar levels and improve your child's focus and attention.

- **Omega-3 fatty acids:** Include sources like fatty fish, flaxseeds, and walnuts to promote brain health and alleviate ADHD symptoms.

- **Minimize processed foods:** Opt for whole, unprocessed options to avoid exacerbating ADHD symptoms.

- **Eliminate food sensitivities:** Identify and eliminate trigger foods from your child's diet to alleviate hyperactivity and inattention.

- **Emphasize nutrient-dense options:** Encourage a variety of fruits, vegetables, whole grains, nuts, seeds, and lean proteins to promote brain health and function.

- **Consistent meal timing:** Establish regular meal schedules to sustain steady energy levels throughout the day.

- **Proper hydration:** Ensure adequate water intake to support cognitive function and overall health.

- **Supplementation:** Under professional guidance, consider supplements like magnesium, zinc, iron, and vitamin D to address deficiencies associated with ADHD symptoms.

- **Behavioral strategies:** Implement routines, clear expectations, positive reinforcement, and dietary changes to establish a holistic treatment plan.

- **Individualized approach:** Collaborating with health care providers and dietitians, tailor nutrition interventions to each child's unique needs and preferences.

As we wrap up this section, you must recognize the insights you have gained. With your new understanding of which foods can exacerbate symptoms of ADHD and which ones can alleviate them, you are equipped with valuable knowledge to make informed decisions for your child's vitality. With dedication and guidance, you can embark on this journey toward better nutrition, setting the stage for your child to thrive and flourish.

Jake's Nutritional Odyssey: Building a Strong Foundation With a Balanced Diet

Jake's journey toward establishing a healthy lifestyle through a balanced diet has been transformative. He began by acknowledging the insights his parents shared with him about the profound influence nutrition could have on managing his most challenging symptoms, including his struggle with listening to instructions in the classroom, his difficulty with organization, and his trouble sitting still.

He got involved with planning meals and allowed his parents to incorporate new tastes and textures slowly. By reducing the intake of his favorite candies and fast-food items and incorporating nutrient-dense foods such as tuna and tofu, greens like spinach and kale, and antioxidants from dark chocolate and strawberries, Jake noticed a remarkable improvement in his hyperactivity and inattention symptoms.

Overall, Jake's experience highlights the lessons of this chapter. His success demonstrates the importance of embracing a balanced diet rich in essential nutrients to manage ADHD and support overall brain health. Through his journey, he has uncovered the transformative power of food as medicine and its profound impact on enhancing cognitive function and well-being.

SUPERFOODS FOR ADHD KIDS

Welcome to the world of superfoods, where delicious meets nutritious, and every bite packs a punch of goodness! In this chapter, you will dive into a topic close to the hearts of many parents like yourself: Superfoods for ADHD kids.

Picture this: A vibrant array of foods bursting with color, flavor, and all the nutrients your child's growing brain needs. We're on a mission to discover the ultimate lineup of superfoods that can help support your child's journey with ADHD, from nutrient-rich veggies to brain-boosting fruits and everything in between.

So, grab a seat at the table as you explore the insights of this chapter and unlock the secrets to nourishing your child's body and mind. Get ready to fuel their adventures with foods that taste amazing and help them thrive! Let us dive into why nutrient-dense foods are the superhero squad for ADHD kids and how they can make a world of difference in your family's daily life.

Let us embrace the power of nutrient-dense foods and give our ADHD kids the nourishment they need to thrive. With creativity and many flavors, we can make every meal a delicious masterpiece!

Superfoods

First up, omega-3 fatty acids. These powerhouse nutrients found in salmon and walnuts are brain boosters on a mission. They are essential for cognitive function, helping to improve focus, memory, and overall brain health. Plus, they can assist in taming ADHD symptoms and keeping them in check.

Next, let us talk about antioxidants. Envision a colorful palette of berries, spinach, and kale. These foods are like the bodyguards of your child's cells, protecting them from damage and inflammation. They can also improve attention span and support better mood regulation, making navigating challenging moments easier.

Don't forget the vitamins! These essential nutrients in familiar favorites, such as vitamin-C-rich oranges and vitamin-D-packed eggs, support your child's overall health and well-being. They are the building blocks of a strong and resilient immune system, keeping sniffles at bay and ensuring your child has the energy to tackle each day with enthusiasm.

But here is the best part: Incorporating nutrient-dense foods into your child's diet does not have to be a chore. You can make mealtimes a fun and exciting adventure for the whole family with delicious food and easy ingredient substitutes. It can be as simple as swapping out processed snacks for crunchy carrots and hummus and trading in sugary cereals for hearty oatmeal topped with fresh berries.

The Power of Nutrient-Dense Foods in Supporting Cognitive Function for Children With ADHD

Let's uncover the vital role of nutrient-dense foods in enhancing cognitive function, especially for children managing hyperactivity and problems with focus. These superhero foods deliver essential nutrients for peak performance and growth.

- **Colorful fruits and vegetables:** Berries, such as blueberries, strawberries, and raspberries, are packed with antioxidants like vitamin C and flavonoids, which help protect brain cells from damage caused by free radicals. Spinach, rich in folate, iron, and vitamin K, supports mental processes and helps maintain brain health. Sweet potatoes are abundant in beta-carotene, a precursor to vitamin A, which plays a crucial role in brain development and function, including memory and learning.

- **Omega-3 fatty acids:** Fatty fish like salmon, mackerel, and trout are excellent sources of omega-3 fatty acids, particularly eicosapentaenoic acid (EPA) and docosahexaenoic acid (DHA). These are essential for brain health, as they contribute to the structure and function of brain cell membranes, promote neuroplasticity, and support neurotransmitter function. Walnuts and flaxseeds are plant-based sources of alpha-linolenic acid (ALA), a precursor to EPA and DHA, which the body can convert into these essential fatty acids. Including omega-3-rich foods in the diet of ADHD children has been associated with improved attention, focus, and behavior.

- **Synergy of nutrients:** Protein-rich foods provide the amino acids necessary for neurotransmitter synthesis, including dopamine and serotonin, which play key roles in mood regulation and cognitive function. Meats like chicken, turkey, and lean beef offer high-quality protein with lower levels of saturated fat. Beans and legumes are protein-rich and provide complex carbohydrates, fiber, and micronutrients like iron and zinc, which are important for energy production and brain health. Almonds, walnuts, peanuts, and other nuts are rich in healthy fats, protein, and antioxidants, and they provide sustained energy throughout the day and support brain function.

Incorporating these superfoods into your child's diet can significantly enhance their focus and attention, and it means providing the fuel for their brains to thrive and succeed in academic and life challenges.

Key Nutrients for ADHD Management

We introduced them at the start of the chapter, but let's now delve deeper into the essential nutrients that have the potential to significantly improve the lives of children with ADHD: omega-3 fatty acids, antioxidants, and vitamins. These nutritional powerhouses are not merely beneficial additions to a diet. They also play a fundamental role in enhancing brain function and fostering overall health.

- **Omega-3 fatty acids:** These vital fats, abundant in foods like fish, nuts, and seeds, play a pivotal role in brain function, assisting in focus, concentration, and mood stability among children with ADHD. Fish varieties such as salmon, mackerel, and sardines stand out as exceptional sources of omega-3 fatty acids, notably EPA and DHA, which are fundamental for brain health. These fatty acids are instrumental in supporting mental functioning, regulating mood, and enhancing attention span, rendering them indispensable components of any ADHD-friendly dietary regimen.

- Antioxidants: Vibrant fruits such as cherries and verdant vegetables like spinach, along with indulgent dark chocolate, boast a wealth of antioxidants crucial for shielding the brain from oxidative stress and inflammation, thereby bolstering the organ's overall health. Berries, including blueberries, strawberries, and raspberries, are veritable powerhouses of antioxidants, as they contain a rich array of vitamin C, flavonoids, and polyphenols. These potent compounds play a pivotal role in safeguarding brain cells from oxidative damage and inflammation, fostering enhanced mental acumen and clarity among children grappling with ADHD.

- **Vitamins:** From the invigorating vitamin C found abundantly in oranges to the enriching vitamin D nestled within eggs, each essential vitamin plays a pivotal role in bolstering brain function and overall well-being, contributing to enhanced mood, immunity, and cognitive prowess. Lush leafy greens like spinach, kale, and Swiss chard stand as true nutritional highflyers, brimming with an array of vital vitamins such as A, C, and K, alongside folate and iron. These essential nutrients are integral to brain health, facilitating neurotransmitter synthesis, bolstering thought processing, and effectively regulating mood.

Incorporating these nutrient superstars into your child's diet doesn't have to be complicated. With simple swaps and creative meal ideas, you can easily ensure they get the nutrients they need to thrive. We'll expand on this later on in this chapter.

Can Nutrition Help Manage Your Child's ADHD Symptoms?

Nutrition serves as a cornerstone in the comprehensive management of ADHD symptoms, playing a pivotal role in supporting not only the alleviation of specific symptoms but also the promotion of overall brain health and function. By providing the body with essential nutrients through a balanced and nourishing diet, you can help your kids experience improvements in cognitive function, mood regulation, and behavioral outcomes.

This holistic approach underscores the importance of incorporating a variety of superfoods, all of which contribute to optimal brain health and function. Moreover, adopting dietary habits that prioritize whole foods while minimizing the intake of processed foods and artificial additives can further enhance the efficacy of nutritional interventions in managing ADHD symptoms and promoting long-term well-being. Here's how:

- **Balancing blood sugar levels:** A balanced diet helps stabilize blood sugar levels, reducing energy crashes and hyperactivity.

- **Supporting brain function:** Nutrient-rich foods provide essential vitamins, minerals, and antioxidants, improving focus, attention, and memory.

- **Reducing potential triggers:** Avoiding foods or additives that trigger ADHD symptoms can minimize their severity.

- **Improving sleep quality:** A nutritious diet contributes to consistent, quality rest, essential for children with ADHD.

- **Enhancing mood and behavior:** Certain nutrients like magnesium and zinc support mood regulation, improving behavior in children with ADHD.

While nutrition isn't a replacement for other treatments, it can significantly alleviate ADHD symptoms when combined with therapy or medication. Consulting with healthcare professionals for personalized guidance is essential.

How Does Diet Affect ADHD in Children?

Diet influences ADHD in several ways:

- **Nutrient intake:** Essential nutrients support optimal brain function, improving focus, attention, and impulse control.

- **Blood sugar levels:** Foods that cause rapid spikes and crashes in blood sugar levels can worsen inattention and hyperactivity.

- **Gut health:** A diet rich in fiber and probiotics supports a healthy gut microbiome, benefiting brain function by facilitating homeostasis and neuroplasticity.

- **Allergens and inflammation:** Inflammatory foods may exacerbate ADHD symptoms in some children.

- **Medication response:** Certain foods may interact with ADHD medications, affecting their efficacy or worsening side effects.

Incorporating a balanced diet filled with whole foods is essential for maintaining good health for everyone. For children with ADHD, though, a healthy diet can also help alleviate their symptoms and improve their overall social, mental, and physical well-being.

Processed foods with high sugar content, artificial dyes, and flavorings have been linked to increased hyperactivity and decreased attention span in children. On the other hand, whole foods such as fruits, vegetables, lean protein, and healthy fats can provide the essential nutrients needed for optimal brain function and support a healthy lifestyle.

Food and Ingredient Substitutions

Let us explore a world of food and ingredient substitutes that can be tailored to children with ADHD. We are diving into how certain artificial ingredients, food additives, and allergens can potentially exacerbate ADHD symptoms in some kids and, more importantly, how to navigate around them.

Picture this: You are in the grocery store, scanning labels and searching for healthier options for your child. But with so many products packed with artificial ingredients and additives, it feels like navigating a minefield. Remember this simple tip to escape this danger zone: Don't buy anything with ingredients you can't pronounce!

And for those of you who have children with dietary restrictions like gluten or dairy intolerances, fear not! There are plenty of options available to accommodate their needs. From gluten-free pasta made from quinoa or brown rice to dairy-free alternatives like almond milk or coconut yogurt, there's no shortage of delicious swaps.

Sugar Substitutions

First off, let us talk about artificial sweeteners. While they may seem like a guilt-free way to satisfy a sweet tooth, they can wreak havoc on ADHD symptoms and health in general. They lead your body to produce insulin in the same way that eating regular sugar does. The problem is that insulin increases hunger and promotes energy stored as fat.

Natural Sweeteners

Instead, use natural sweeteners like honey, maple syrup, and pureed dates. These options are preferable because they add sweetness without harmful side effects and provide additional nutrients and antioxidants.

Dates are high in fiber, which is excellent for gut health, as soluble fiber helps keep cholesterol low. They are also a great source of potassium, phosphorus, calcium, and magnesium. Additionally, they are high in antioxidants, including flavonoids, carotenoids, and phenolic acid, which can lower the risks of diabetes, dementia, heart disease, and cancer. Regularly consuming dates may also improve brain power, memory, and learning. You can puree Medjool dates and add them to oatmeal or incorporate them into a shake with oat or almond milk, hemp seeds, ice, and cinnamon.

Maple syrup contains nutrients such as manganese, riboflavin, zinc, magnesium, calcium, and potassium. An additional benefit to this ingredient is that it won't spike your blood sugar levels as quickly as plain sugar will. It also contains antioxidants and supports gut health by preventing inflammation and promoting prebiotic activity.

Honey has antibacterial and antioxidant properties that protect against infections and other diseases. It also contains vitamins and minerals, including calcium, potassium, vitamin C, zinc, phenolic acids, and flavonoids. This sweetener also feeds the beneficial bacteria in your gut. It is better at soothing a sore throat than cough suppressants and drops, making it an excellent ingredient to keep around.

Breakfast Substitutions

Let's also talk about breakfast substitutions. Half of all Americans eat cereal for breakfast, a processed food filled with sugar. So, what are some alternative breakfast options?

Whether cooked on the stove or instant, oatmeal is a classic and a firm favorite. Overnight oats, in particular, are a super easy option that can be changed daily by incorporating different toppings.

Like overnight oats, chia pudding is versatile and straightforward to make. The day before you want to eat it, mix chia seeds with non-dairy milk and let it chill in the refrigerator overnight.

Then there is yogurt mixed with granola—preferably homemade so you can control the amount of sugar that goes into it. Smoothies are another great way to pack in fruits, vegetables, and nuts, especially when you and your child run late in the morning.

Finally, cooked breakfast options include a tofu, egg scramble, and avocado toast for a quick but wholesome bite.

Choosing a Healthier Bread Option

To choose healthier bread options, keep the following tips in mind when making substitutions:

- Look for "whole grain" on the label. In more processed flours, the nutrients and fiber-rich parts of the grain are removed. So, the less interference, the better.

- Check the label to ensure you get 3–5 grams of fiber per serving.

- Sugar is usually added to bread to delay staling, so avoid those with added sweetening agents such as molasses, cane sugar, and tapioca syrup.

- Look for other refined flours, including tapioca starch, maltodextrin, and white rice flour.

- Avoid long ingredient lists containing lots of additives.

- Avoid high sodium content; there should be no more than 160 mg per slice.

- Look for the protein content on the label. Whole grains are solid sources of plant proteins, and you should ideally get 3 grams of the macronutrient per slice.

Next-Level Breads

- **Sprouted bread:** Sprouted grain offers more nutritional value than mature alternatives and is made with whole grains that have been allowed to germinate. This process increases the bioavailability and absorbability of the nutrients, and it also helps degrade antinutrients like phytic acid, which can inhibit the absorption of minerals like iron.

- **Seeded bread:** Seeds contain fiber, protein, unsaturated fats, which are the good kind, and vitamins and minerals.

- **Rye bread:** Rye has a lower glycemic index than wheat, so it has less impact on blood sugar. It also contains impressive amounts of vitamins and minerals, helping to maintain healthy immune systems, metabolism, and energy levels.

- **Sourdough bread:** This bread is made using a fermented starter that has its own microbiome. Whole-grain sourdough breads are associated with a lower risk of heart disease, diabetes, and cancer.

So, the next time you are grocery shopping, remember these tips. Now that your knowledge base has expanded feel free to get creative with your swaps. Your child's health and happiness are worth it!

What Healthy Snacks Are Suitable for Children With ADHD to Include in Their Diet?

ADHD can cause children to struggle with focus, organization, and impulsivity. By providing healthy snacks rich in protein, fiber, and complex carbohydrates, you can help them maintain a consistent energy level throughout the day and support their mental functioning.

Instead of reaching for processed snacks loaded with artificial flavors and preservatives, opt for healthier alternatives like fresh fruit, veggies with hummus, or homemade trail mix. These options provide a satisfying crunch without the unwanted additives, keeping your child fueled and focused throughout the day. Other great inclusions are fresh fruits and vegetables, nuts and seeds, low-fat dairy products, and whole-grain crackers or bread. These choices will not only nourish your child's body, but they can also help them stay more alert and focused during school or other activities. Here are some nutritious options:

- **Fresh fruit:** Sliced apples, berries, grapes, oranges, and bananas are convenient and packed with vitamins, minerals, and fiber. Combine them with nut butter or yogurt for added protein and healthy fats.

- **Vegetable sticks:** Carrot sticks, cucumber slices, bell pepper strips, and cherry tomatoes make for crunchy snacks that are rich in antioxidants and fiber. Serve them with hummus or guacamole for extra flavor and nutrition.

- **Trail mix:** Create a homemade trail mix with nuts, seeds, dried fruits, and whole-grain cereal. This combination provides protein, healthy fats, and complex carbohydrates for sustained energy.

- **Greek yogurt:** High in protein and calcium, supporting brain health and muscle function. Go for a plain variety and add fresh fruit, honey, or a drizzle of maple syrup for natural sweetness.

- **Hard-boiled eggs:** Hard-boiled eggs are portable, protein-rich snacks that help stabilize blood sugar levels and promote satiety. Sprinkle them with a pinch of salt and pepper for flavor.

- **Cheese and whole grain crackers:** Pair sliced cheese with whole grain crackers for a satisfying protein, calcium, and complex carbohydrates snack.

- **Popcorn:** Air-popped popcorn is a whole-grain snack that is low in calories and high in fiber. Sprinkle salt or nutritional yeast on top for enhanced taste.

- **Smoothies:** Blend fresh or frozen fruits, leafy greens, Greek yogurt, and a splash of milk for a nutrient-packed snack that's easy to customize.

- **Homemade energy balls:** These no-bake treats are perfect for on-the-go snacking and can be made using oats, nut butter, honey, and mix-ins like dried fruit, seeds, or dark chocolate chips.

- **Whole grain toast:** Top toasted bread with avocado, mashed banana, nut butter, or cottage cheese for a quick and nutritious snack loaded with fiber and healthy fats.

Incorporating these ADHD-friendly snacks into your child's diet gives them the sustained energy and essential nutrients they need to support their concentration and overall well-being.

The most important thing to remember is to read labels carefully and be mindful of what you put into your child's body. Make informed decisions and opt for whole, nutrient-dense foods whenever possible.

Jake's Journey: Harnessing the Power of Superfoods to Manage ADHD Symptoms

Jake's exploration of superfoods has been enlightening for other kids with ADHD. He discovered that certain foods rich in nutrients like omega-3 fatty acids, antioxidants, and vitamins can help him manage his symptoms significantly.

By incorporating more superfoods such as avocado, broccoli, eggs, sweet potatoes, and almonds into his diet, Jake noticed a remarkable improvement in his ADHD symptoms. These nutrient-dense foods helped him manage his restlessness and inattention. They supported his overall brain health and cognitive function, helping him feel better and enhancing his academic performance.

Jake's mom exemplified the process of incorporating superfoods into the whole family's diet by crafting specific meal plans that highlighted supercharged macro- and micronutrients. By infusing creativity and delightful recipes into their meals, she empowered Jake and the rest of his family to realize their full potential and embrace life to the fullest.

REDUCING SUGAR AND ARTIFICIAL ADDITIVES

Sugar and artificial additives! These troublemakers can wreak havoc on your kids' health and behavior. To help you overcome this hurdle to a healthier diet, we have the ultimate guide to help you become a label-reading superhero and uncover hidden sugars like a pro.

First, grab your magnifying glasses and get ready to decode food labels. Look out for tricky aliases like "high-fructose corn syrup" and "dextrose," lurking in everything from cereals to sauces. By arming yourself with this knowledge, you can steer clear of these sugar traps and make informed choices for your family.

What about those sudden sugar cravings that we all sometimes experience? Worry not! This chapter will give you strategies to help tame those urges and satisfy your kids without dipping into a sugar overload. From swapping processed snacks for nourishing alternatives to adding more protein and fiber into your child's meals, we have plenty of tricks to help you navigate the sugar and additive maze.

So, the next time you are stocking up on groceries, keep your eyes peeled for artificial imposters and arm yourself with the tools to make healthier choices for your family. With some know-how and determination, you can conquer the sugar monster and set your kids on the road to a healthier, happier future.

What Sugar and Artificial Additives Do to a Child With ADHD

Let's delve into the detrimental consequences of excessive sugar consumption and the adverse effects that artificial additives commonly found in processed foods can have.

By outlining how sugar interacts with the brain and influences ADHD symptoms, we aim to shed light on the importance of dietary interventions in managing ADHD. By engaging in this discussion, you will gain valuable insights into the role of nutrition in supporting your child's well-being and learn practical strategies for minimizing their exposure to these harmful substances. So, let us venture together on this road to understanding as we explore the complex relationship between diet and ADHD symptomatology.

We have already established that excessive sugar consumption and artificial additives can have significant effects on children with ADHD, but it's worth exploring why that is.

- **Sugar:** Elevated intake can trigger rapid shifts in blood sugar levels, leading to abrupt energy dips and mood swings. In children with ADHD, these fluctuations can exacerbate symptoms such as hyperactivity, impulsivity, and difficulty concentrating. Additionally, sugary foods often lack essential nutrients, further contributing to nutritional deficiencies that may impact brain function and behavior.

- **Artificial additives:** Synthetic ingredients like colorings, flavor enhancers, and preservatives are frequently present in processed foods and snacks. These additives have been linked to disruptions in neurotransmitter function in the brain, potentially worsening ADHD symptoms. Studies suggest that certain artificial additives may increase hyperactivity and impulsivity in children with ADHD, making it challenging for them to focus and regulate their behavior effectively (Arnold et al., 2012).

Overall, reducing your child's sugar intake may help alleviate ADHD symptoms and improve their overall well-being. By opting for whole, nutrient-rich foods and minimizing the consumption of processed snacks and sugary treats, you can support your child's health and manage their ADHD more effectively.

Understanding the Effects of Sugar on Children With ADHD

Prepare to discover the intricate relationship between sugar, artificial additives, and ADHD in children. Let us delve into the multifaceted impacts of these substances, which compelling insights from scientific research have supported. With this knowledge, you can make informed decisions about your child's nutrition.

This proactive approach helps stabilize their blood sugar levels, promotes sustained energy, and reduces reliance on artificial additives that disrupt brain function. Incorporating fresh fruits, vegetables, lean proteins, and whole grains into your child's diet provides essential nutrients to support their focus, self-regulation, and overall well-being.

- **Reduce sugar intake:** By minimizing the consumption of sugary treats like candies, sodas, and desserts, as well as processed snacks laden with hidden sugars, you can mitigate the risk of rapid blood sugar spikes followed by crashes. These fluctuations can trigger mood swings, irritability, and difficulty concentrating for your child.

- **Limit artificial additives:** Steering clear of foods that contain artificial colors, flavor enhancers, and preservatives is crucial in safeguarding the neurological health of children with ADHD.

- **Artificial flavorings:** These chemical compounds, used to mimic natural flavors or enhance existing ones, are frequently listed simply as "artificial flavors" in ingredient lists.

- **Preservatives:** Chemical substances such as butylated hydroxyanisole (BHA) and butylated hydroxytoluene (BHT) are added to food to prevent spoilage and extend shelf life.

- **Sweeteners:** Artificial sweeteners like aspartame, saccharin, and sucralose are commonly added to foods and beverages to provide sweetness without adding calories.

- **Monosodium glutamate (MSG):** This flavor enhancer is often added to savory dishes, soups, and snacks to enhance taste.

- **Trans fats:** Artificial trans fats, often listed as "partially hydrogenated oils," are used to improve processed foods' texture and shelf life but are harmful to health when consumed in excess.

Promoting Awareness and Determination

We, as parents, can collaborate to raise awareness about the impact of diet on ADHD symptoms and advocate for healthier dietary choices in our community. By sharing knowledge and resources, we can create a supportive environment that empowers other parents to help their children manage ADHD symptoms and promote our children's well-being and success.

Let us unite to fight against sugar crashes and artificial ingredients! With awareness and determination, we can pave the way for a brighter, more balanced future for children with this neurodevelopmental disorder. By making informed dietary choices, we can positively impact our children's health and well-being, fostering a supportive environment for their journey toward improved attention and focus.

Learning to Read Food Labels and Identify Hidden Sugars

As the parent of a child with ADHD, managing your child's dietary intake plays a pivotal role in promoting their optimal wellness. Learning to read food labels and identify hidden sugars equips you with the confidence to make informed choices that support your child's unique needs. By examining ingredient lists and nutritional information, you can steer clear of foods containing excessive sugars, artificial additives, and preservatives, all of which can exacerbate hyperactivity and difficulty with focus.

Taking a proactive approach empowers parents to prioritize whole, nutrient-rich foods that provide essential vitamins, minerals, and antioxidants crucial for cognitive function and emotional regulation. Additionally, reducing sugar can help children develop healthy appetite regulation, influence their taste preferences, and improve their learning ability and memory. Through ongoing education and advocacy, you can create a supportive environment that fosters your child's success in managing ADHD symptoms.

Here is why it is crucial, as well as some tips to help you navigate food labels effectively:

- **Understanding hidden sugars:** Hidden sugars lurk in numerous processed foods, even those with no overt sweetness. These agents contribute to blood sugar fluctuations, thereby worsening ADHD symptoms like impulsivity and hyperactivity. Being mindful of them is crucial for managing ADHD effectively.

- **Impact on ADHD symptoms:** Consuming foods that are high in hidden sugars can contribute to mood swings, irritability, and difficulty concentrating in children with ADHD. By learning to identify and limit hidden sugars in their diet, you can help manage your child's symptoms more effectively.

- **Reading food labels:** When reading food labels, look for terms like:

    - sucrose

    - high-fructose corn syrup

    - corn syrup solids

    - fructose

    - glucose

- dextrose

- molasses

- cane sugar

- invert sugar

- brown rice syrup

- agave nectar

These are all added sugars that may be hiding in packaged foods.

- **Checking ingredient lists:** Ingredients on food labels are listed by weight, so if sugar is among the first few ingredients, the product likely contains significant added sugars. However, with over 200 terms used for sugar, companies can also place them lower on the label, but the individual listings still contribute to overall intake.

- **Comparing products:** When choosing between similar products, compare the nutrition labels to see which contains less added sugars. Opt for products with lower sugar content or choose unsweetened alternatives whenever possible.

- **Considering alternative names:** Remember that sugar can hide behind various names on food labels, so you must familiarize yourself with the different terms used to describe them.

- **Limiting processed foods:** To reduce hidden-sugar intake, prioritize whole, unprocessed foods such as fruits, vegetables, lean proteins, whole grains, and dairy products without added sugars. Cooking meals from scratch allows you to control the ingredients and avoid the harmful ingredients commonly found in processed foods.

Foods to Steer Clear of if Your Child Has ADHD

When using dietary interventions to address ADHD symptoms in children, it is crucial to be attentive to specific foods that could potentially worsen their symptoms. Here are some foods to avoid or limit:

- **Sugar and sweets:** Excessive consumption of sugary foods like candies, sodas, and desserts can lead to energy crashes and worsen hyperactivity and impulsivity.

- **Artificial additives:** Foods containing synthetic dyes, flavor enhancers, and preservatives, commonly found in snacks like cookies and flavored crackers, can disrupt neurotransmitter function and exacerbate ADHD symptoms.

- **Highly processed foods:** Processed foods like ready meals and tinned products that are high in unhealthy fats, refined sugars, and additives may contribute to inflammation and oxidative stress, potentially worsening ADHD symptoms.

- **Fast food and junk food:** High-calorie, low-nutrient foods like fast-food burgers, fries, and savory snacks like potato chips offer little nutritional value and may contribute to behavioral problems and hyperactivity.

- **Caffeine:** While small quantities of caffeine might enhance focus in particular children, excessive consumption can result in jitteriness, irritability, and disrupted sleep, exacerbating symptoms such as difficulty with organization, and it can cause increased anxiety.

Minimizing or avoiding these foods and focusing on a diet rich in the alternatives we have suggested throughout this book can better support your child's overall health and well-being while effectively managing their ADHD symptoms.

Implementing Strategies for Reducing Sugar Cravings in Children

Alright, parents, it is time to tackle those sugar cravings head-on and regain control of our child's diet! Implementing practical strategies and techniques can empower you and your child to make healthier choices and minimize your response to the allure of sugary snacks. Let us continue toward improved health and wellness for our families!

Here are some practical strategies and techniques to help reduce those irresistible urges for all things sweet:

- **Embrace fiber:** Where can we find this indigestible carb? Fruits, vegetables, and whole grains. Fiber plays a vital role in slowing digestion, leading to prolonged feelings of fullness and aiding in curbing cravings. Additionally, it fuels the gut microbiome, promoting a healthy and balanced digestive system.

- **Choose natural sweeteners:** Consider using naturally sweet foods. Artificial alternatives like sucralose and aspartame have effects similar to regular sugar on the body. They still lead to insulin release, promoting energy stored as fat and increasing the hunger response. Naturally sweet foods like fruit have fiber to slow down the digestion of natural sugars, generating less insulin production.

- **Gradual reduction:** Implementing change gradually to ease the transition and make it more sustainable for you and your child. Week by week, reduce the amount of added sugar in your child's diet and replace it with healthier alternatives.

- **Lead by example:** Be a role model for your child by demonstrating healthy eating habits yourself. Show them that nutritious foods can be delicious and satisfying and involve them in meal planning and preparation to foster a positive relationship with food.

- **Stay consistent:** Consistency plays a vital role in reducing sugar cravings. Stick to your plan and be patient, as it may take time for your child's taste preferences to adjust to a lower-sugar diet.

- **Address underlying factors:** Sometimes, sugar cravings are triggered by stress, boredom, or emotional eating. If your child expresses hunger, let them wait 15 minutes before indulging them. During that time, encourage them to explore alternative coping mechanisms such as participating in physical activity, practicing relaxation techniques, or expressing themselves through creative outlets. These strategies can help them manage triggers without resorting to sugary foods.

Avoid implementing drastic changes overnight! The human body tends to resist sudden, significant shifts. Instead, opt for gradual adjustments. Small steps pave the way for lasting alterations in tastes and habits, fostering lifelong healthy changes. Show patience and offer unwavering support as you collaborate with experts and as a family to craft a balanced and nutritious diet tailored to overcome the challenges of ADHD. With dedication and persistence, you can guide your child through sugar cravings and instill enduring healthy eating habits that will benefit them for years to come.

Sugar and ADHD in Kids: What's the Connection?

The relationship between sugar consumption and ADHD in children is a widely discussed and debated topic that has garnered significant attention in both research endeavors and public discourse. Experts have conducted extensive studies and dedicated considerable effort to investigating the potential link between sugar intake and ADHD symptoms, aiming to elucidate the impact of dietary factors on neurodevelopment and behavior in children.

The complex interplay between sugar consumption, brain function, and ADHD manifestations has fueled ongoing scientific inquiry, leading to a wealth of studies exploring various facets of this relationship. As our understanding continues to evolve, ongoing research seeks to shed light on the nuanced interactions between dietary habits, neurobiological mechanisms, and ADHD symptomatology, providing valuable insights for us parents, clinicians, and educators alike.

While sugar itself doesn't cause ADHD, there are several ways in which it can impact symptoms and behavior:

- **Blood sugar spikes and crashes:** The rapid consumption of sugary foods or drinks can lead to sharp spikes and subsequent drops in children's blood sugar levels. These fluctuations can trigger changes in energy levels and mood, potentially worsening symptoms of ADHD like hyperactivity, impulsivity, and difficulty concentrating. While research results regarding the impact of sugar intake on ADHD symptoms vary, some studies have found a correlation between increased sugar consumption and heightened hyperactivity and impulsivity in children with the disorder. However, other studies have not established a significant association.

- **Blood sugar levels:** Consuming sugary foods can result in fluctuations in blood sugar levels, which can lead to alterations in energy levels and mood. While these shifts may not directly cause ADHD, they can exacerbate symptoms such as hyperactivity and inattention.

- **Influence on neurotransmitters:** Excessive sugar consumption has been implicated in disrupting the balance of neurotransmitters in the brain, notably dopamine and serotonin, which play key roles in mood and behavior regulation. Imbalances in these neurotransmitters are associated with ADHD symptoms. Sugar intake can impact the activity of dopamine and serotonin, influencing mood and behavior regulation.

- **Inflammation:** Excessive sugar consumption has been linked to increased inflammation in the body, which can potentially impact brain function and worsen ADHD symptoms. Chronic inflammation is associated with various health issues, including cognitive impairment and behavioral challenges.

- **Dietary patterns:** Children with diets high in sugar and processed foods often lack essential nutrients crucial for brain health and function. Conversely, adopting a diet rich in nutrient-dense foods such as fruits, vegetables, whole grains, and lean proteins may help alleviate ADHD symptoms—a fact we have emphasized throughout this book. These foods provide vital vitamins, minerals, and antioxidants that support overall brain health and function.

It is important to note that the relationship between sugar and ADHD is complex, and individual responses may vary. While some kids may be more sensitive to sugar and experience worsened symptoms, others may not be as affected. Additionally, sugar intake should be considered within the context of overall dietary patterns and lifestyle factors.

Adopting a balanced diet that limits added sugars and emphasizes whole, nutritious foods is beneficial for overall health and may help manage inattention and hyperactive behavior in kids. Seeking advice from a health care professional, like a pediatrician or registered dietitian, can offer personalized guidance and recommendations for managing ADHD through nutrition.

Sugar-Free Success: Jake's Journey to Healthier Eating Transforms His Family Dynamics

Jake's success in reducing sugar in his diet was a personal victory and a transformative experience for his entire family. Initially, Jake's diet mirrored that of many children: It was abundant in sugary snacks and processed foods. However, as his parents became aware of the harmful effects of excessive sugar intake, they embarked on a gradual journey to overhaul his diet.

Jake initially resisted the changes, as he was accustomed to the allure of sugary treats. Yet, with patient encouragement from his parents, he gradually embraced healthier alternatives. As his intake of these snacks diminished, Jake's behavior transformed. He exhibited increased focus and attentiveness, accompanied by fewer instances of unrestrained movement, outbursts, and mood swings. As they observed improvements in his overall mood and energy levels, his parents were encouraged to continue their efforts.

Over time, Jake's palate adapted to the healthier offerings. He developed a preference for the more nutritious foods he was offered. His parents introduced him to diverse fruits and vegetables, which he grew to enjoy. With reduced hidden-sugar intake and the inclusion of nutrient-dense foods, Jake continued to exhibit positive behavioral changes. He became more engaged in schoolwork, excelled academically, and demonstrated enhanced emotional regulation.

Through gradual sugar reduction and emphasizing wholesome nutrition, Jake and his family fostered positive developments that supported his health and well-being, strengthened familial bonds, and instilled lifelong habits for a healthier future.

The Gut-Brain Connection: Healing the Gut for Improved Attention

Have you ever wondered how your stomach and your brain are connected? The relationship is like a stable friendship. When both parties are happy, your child can learn and have fun daily. So, in this chapter, we will explore how helping your child take care of their tummy can sharpen their brain, especially when it comes to paying attention and being better learners.

Grab your explorer hats and prepare for an adventure-packed quest to discover the secrets of healing the gut for super-powered attention!

Discovering the Gut Microbiome

Did you know healing an unbalanced gut microbiome with prebiotics can help improve attention and behavior? It is true! Let us unpack this exciting discovery together.

Imagine your gut microbiome as a busy city, bustling with bacteria similar to tiny workers who play a significant role in the brain's work, mainly when focusing and being well-behaved. By feeding your stomach the right food, like prebiotics, you can help these friendly organisms flourish and balance the systems they oversee.

Now, let us talk about prebiotics. They are like the superheroes of the food world, fueling and strengthening the good bacteria in the gut. Foods like bananas, oats, garlic, and onions are packed with them and are ready to give your digestive tract the boost it needs to support your brain.

In addition to prebiotics, another essential component for gut health is probiotics. These microorganisms can fortify the gut by improving it and restoring the good bacteria that may be lost due to various causes. They can also help ensure a healthy balance between good and bad bacteria.

By teaching your child to pay attention to what they eat and how their belly feels after eating, you can help them discover if certain ones disagree with them. Children should understand that some foods can make their stomachs feel funny and may affect how they pay attention or behave. By encouraging them to determine which foods are good for their digestion and which disrupts it, you can help them better manage their behavioral and concentration difficulties.

So, let us lead by example and join forces with our stomachs. Enjoy delicious prebiotic and probiotic-packed foods, and help our children become the ultimate attention and behavior champions. With a bit of detective work and some tasty, gut-friendly treats, there is no adventure we can't conquer.

Unlocking the Gut-Brain Connection: How Tummy Health Shapes ADHD Symptoms in Kids

While we know that ADHD is something many kids deal with, we are constantly learning more about the disorder and how to manage it. Recent research has shown that there might be a link between ADHD and gut health, and experts are saying children's tummies might have something to do with the development and manifestation of the disorder. Although scientists are still figuring out all the details, it seems like the gut might play a significant role in how ADHD shows up in our kids.

So, why do some experts think the stomach matters? They say it's because of the gut microbiome—a bustling city of bacteria living inside us. Studies have found that when this city gets out of balance, it can cause inflammation, which can negatively impact the brain and worsen ADHD symptoms.

Here are some things to think about:

- **Microbiome imbalance:** Our digestive tracts are home to tons of bacteria that help digest food, keeping us healthy and affecting how our brains work. Some studies have shown that kids with ADHD might have different kinds of bacteria living in their tummies than kids without the disorder, meaning their microbiome "neighborhoods" might be different (Kids, 2023).

- **Inflammation and immune response:** When our stomachs are out of balance, it can lead to inflammation and impair the immune system. Inflammation might affect the brain, too, making ADHD symptoms feel even trickier to deal with for affected children.

- **Nutrient absorption:** Our gut is where we get all the good stuff from our food, like the vitamins and minerals that keep our brains sharp. But if the balance between healthy and unhealthy bacteria is off-kilter, we might not get all the necessary nutrients.

- **Food sensitivities:** Like most of us, our children might have tummies that don't respond well to certain foods. Things like artificial additives, preservatives, gluten, or dairy might bother them more than they do other children. Cutting back on these foods might help some kids feel better.

- **Stress and anxiety:** When we're feeling stressed or anxious, it can also mess with our gut microbiome. And children who have got ADHD might be more likely to feel this way, which can create a loop of tummy troubles and feeling overwhelmed.

What can we do about it? Some experts think caring for the gut with good food and healthy habits might help with ADHD symptoms. However, talking to a doctor or healthcare professional is essential before significantly changing a diet or treatment plan. They can give you the best advice based on what your child needs.

And hey, let's not forget the awesome adventure of helping our children understand how their tummies and brains work together! With science as our guide, we can unlock the power of a healthy stomach and encourage them to reach for the stars. When their guts and brains are working together, there's no limit to what they can achieve.

Exploring the Connection Between Gut Health and ADHD Symptoms

Let us explore the intriguing connection between gut health and attention levels, particularly concerning children with ADHD.

A busy metropolis of bacteria influences brain function inside our tummies, affecting attention and energy levels. When good and bad gut bacteria are imbalanced, attention can suffer, and hyperactivity can disrupt the gut-brain connection. But fear not! Scientists have uncovered ways to restore this balance, promoting focus and control. We can achieve boundless potential with their findings and a sense of adventure!

For one, we support gut health and enhance brain function by nurturing our bellies with foods like fruits, veggies, and probiotics. A harmonious gut sends positive signals to the brain, aiding focus and calmness. Together, the two form a superhero duo, empowering us to be our best selves.

The connection between gut health and ADHD symptoms is a topic of growing interest in scientific research. Here are some critical aspects of this connection:

- **Gut microbiome's impact on kids' ADHD behavior:** The difference in gut microbiome composition can significantly affect brain function and children's behavior, especially those with ADHD. Alterations in gut bacteria may lead to inflammation, immune system imbalance, and disrupted neurotransmitter production, contributing to symptoms like hyperactivity and difficulty concentrating. Recognizing this link highlights the importance of addressing digestive health through dietary and lifestyle interventions to improve ADHD management beyond conventional approaches.

- **Dietary factors:** Diet plays a significant role in shaping the gut microbiome. Specific nutritional patterns, such as high-sugar, high-fat, and low-fiber diets, can promote dysbiosis and inflammation, potentially worsening hyperactivity and symptoms associated with trouble with concentration. Conversely, fiber-rich diets and regularly consuming prebiotics and probiotics may support a healthy digestive tract and mitigate ADHD symptoms.

- **Inflammation and immune function:** Dysbiosis, characterized by an imbalance in the gut microbiota, can result in heightened intestinal permeability and systemic inflammation. Chronic inflammation and dysregulated immune responses have been implicated in the pathophysiology of ADHD. Immune activation in the gut can trigger inflammatory signals that impact brain function and may exacerbate the disorder's symptoms.

- **Neurotransmitter production:** The gut microbiota is critical in synthesizing neurotransmitters such as serotonin, dopamine, and gamma-aminobutyric acid (GABA), vital for regulating mood, cognition, and behavior. Alterations in the gut microbiome composition can affect neurotransmitter production, potentially contributing to ADHD symptoms.

- **Gut-brain axis:** The brain and the gut are linked via a bidirectional communication network called the gut-brain axis. Through it, they communicate via various pathways, including neural, immune, and hormonal signaling. Changes in the stomach's microbiome can influence these pathways and subsequently impact brain function and behavior.

The correlation between gut health and ADHD symptoms highlights the significance of the gut microbiome as a potential focus for therapeutic interventions in managing the condition. Additional research is warranted to comprehensively grasp the mechanisms underpinning this relationship and devise targeted interventions to promote gut health and alleviate symptoms.

Unraveling Food Sensitivities and ADHD: A Comprehensive Guide

The intriguing world of food and its profound impact on children's superpowers, particularly those with ADHD, is worth discovering. In this section, you will learn the hidden truths about food sensitivities and how they influence behavior, attention, and hyperactivity levels.

In our brief discussion earlier in this chapter, you learned that your body can act as a sidekick to you as a detective, presenting clear clues about how various foods affect you. Some of them play the role of sneaky villains, disrupting focus and energy levels, especially for kids with ADHD.

By teaching your child to acknowledge their body's cues, you can help them actively participate as an investigator and work with them to identify common troublemakers such as artificial colors, preservatives, and certain sugars. Once you've detained the guilty parties, you can swap them out for healthier options like fresh fruits, veggies, and whole grains to restore balance in the body and mind.

Understanding Common Food Sensitivities Associated With ADHD:

- **Gluten:** Found in wheat, barley, rye, and processed foods, gluten can induce food sensitivity or celiac disease, which can exacerbate ADHD symptoms.

- **Dairy:** Lactose and casein proteins in dairy products may trigger digestive issues and inflammation, leading to behavioral changes in some children with ADHD.

- **Food additives:** Artificial colors, flavors, and preservatives commonly found in processed foods have been linked to hyperactivity and other ADHD symptoms.

- **Sugar:** While not universal, some children may experience increased hyperactivity and difficulty concentrating after consuming sugary foods and beverages.

- **Salicylates:** These are naturally occurring compounds in certain fruits, veggies, and spices that might induce behavioral changes in individuals with salicylate sensitivities and who also have ADHD.

The impact of these food sensitivities on a child's behavior can vary widely. While some children may experience noticeable improvements in focus and behavior after eliminating trigger foods, others may not exhibit significant changes. Identifying and avoiding potential food sensitivities through structured approaches like elimination diets or sensitivity testing can help you manage your child's ADHD symptoms more effectively.

Navigating the Journey of Identifying and Eliminating Trigger Foods:

- **Keep a food diary:** Tracking your child's daily intake and any associated changes in behavior or symptoms to identify patterns. Our accompanying workbook helps you keep track of your child's foods and drinks.

- **Observe patterns:** Look for correlations between specific foods and your child's ADHD symptoms, paying attention to consistent behavior changes.

- **Consider common triggers:** Be mindful of common trigger foods, such as gluten, dairy, artificial additives, sugar, and salicylates.

- **Implement an elimination diet:** Work with health care professionals to remove potential trigger foods for a specified period and gradually reintroduce them while monitoring your child's reactions.

- **Focus on whole foods:** Prioritize nutrient-dense foods like fruits, vegetables, lean proteins, whole grains, and healthy fats to support overall health and mitigate ADHD symptoms.

Every child is unique, so what works for one may not work for another. With patience, careful observation, and professional guidance, you can successfully identify and eliminate trigger foods, reduce ADHD symptoms, and promote your child's overall well-being.

Unlocking the Power of Nutrition: Implementing an Elimination Diet for Managing ADHD Symptoms

Incorporating an elimination diet can be beneficial for children with ADHD and their families. Here's how you can integrate it into the meal plan:

Implementing an Elimination Diet

Week 1-4: The Preparation Phase

- Ensure that you provide a variety of colorful fruits and vegetables to maximize your child's nutrient intake.

- Incorporate lean proteins like poultry, fish, tofu, and legumes to support brain health.

- For sustained energy levels, offer whole grains like quinoa, brown rice, and oats.

- Encourage hydration with plenty of water throughout the day.

- Adjust portion sizes based on your child's age, appetite, and activity level.

- Consider involving your child in meal planning and preparation to foster independence and promote a positive relationship with food.

Week 5–9: Elimination Phase

- During these weeks, focus on eliminating the five most common triggering foods associated with ADHD symptoms: artificial additives, food colorings, preservatives, dairy, and gluten.

- Emphasize whole, minimally processed foods such as fruits, vegetables, lean proteins, nuts, seeds, and gluten-free grains.

- Read food labels carefully and choose products free from artificial additives, colorings, and preservatives. Opt for dairy alternatives like almond milk or coconut yogurt, and choose gluten-free grains like quinoa, brown rice, or oats.

- Keep a detailed journal to track behavior, mood changes, and any noticeable improvements or worsening of symptoms during this phase. This can help identify potential trigger foods.

Week 10–14: Reintroduction Phase

- Gradually reintroduce one eliminated food at a time, separated by one to two weeks, to observe how each food affects your child's behavior and mood.

- Start with small amounts of the reintroduced food and monitor the response for any adverse reactions or changes in your child's symptoms.

- Continue journaling and note any differences in behavior or mood after reintroducing each food.

- After reincorporating all five food types, analyze your journal entries to identify patterns or correlations between specific foods and ADHD symptoms.

Tips for Success:
- **Preparation:** Plan your child's meals and snacks in advance to ensure their compliance with the elimination diet. Stock up on alternative ingredients and snacks to avoid your child giving in to temptation.

- **Communication:** Keep open communication with health care professionals, such as pediatricians or dietitians, for guidance and support.

- **Family involvement:** Involve your partner and other household members to create a supportive environment and encourage your child to keep going.

- **Education:** Share your newfound knowledge about the purpose of the elimination diet with your child and involve them in food choices and decision-making to empower them to manage their ADHD symptoms.

By incorporating an elimination diet in your child's meal plan, you can gain valuable insights into how food affects their behavior and mood. This will ultimately help them make informed decisions about their diet and better manage their ADHD symptoms as they grow and mature.

Implementing Gut-Healing Protocols and Incorporating Prebiotics for Digestive Health

You are now ready to unlock the secrets of gut-healing magic and boost your child's digestive health while supercharging their attention. First, let us dive into prebiotics—the unsung heroes of gut health. These magical substances are fertilizer for good gut bacteria, restoring balance and promoting a healthier body. Join your child in loading up on prebiotic-rich foods like bananas, oats, garlic, and onions to support the digestive tract's well-being.

Lifestyle changes are also crucial, so prioritize sleep, hydration, and regular exercise for your whole family. Together with consuming prebiotics, you should all embrace a rainbow of nutritious foods for gut-healing greatness. By doing this, you will help your child conquer any obstacle with a happy tummy, laser-focused mind, and a sprinkle of magic and determination.

Implementing gut-healing protocols and incorporating prebiotics for digestive health in children with ADHD involves several practical strategies:

- **Dietary modifications:** Adopting a gut-friendly diet rich in whole, unprocessed foods is crucial. Encourage your child to consume fiber-rich fruits and vegetables, whole grains, and lean proteins. Limit or eliminate processed foods, refined sugars, and artificial additives, which can disrupt digestive health.

- **Probiotic supplementation:** Consider incorporating probiotic supplements into your child's daily routine. They can help alleviate ADHD-related digestive issues and promote gut health. Look for high-quality versions that have been specifically formulated for children.

- **Prebiotic-rich foods:** Introduce prebiotic-rich foods to nourish beneficial gut bacteria in your child's diet. Examples include walnuts, chickpeas, chia seeds, shallots, broccoli, and brown rice. These foods contain non-digestible fibers that promote the growth of healthy gut bacteria.

- **Fermented foods:** Incorporate fermented foods like yogurt, kefir, sauerkraut, kimchi, miso, and kombucha into your child's diet. These foods contain beneficial probiotics that can contribute to a healthy gut microbiome.

- **Hydration:** Remind your child to drink plenty of water throughout the day to ensure they stay adequately hydrated. Proper hydration supports digestive health by aiding in the transportation of nutrients and the elimination of waste products.

- **Stress management:** Chronic stress can adversely affect gut health, underscoring the importance of cultivating a supportive and stress-free environment. Help your child manage pressure by guiding them through relaxation techniques and mindfulness practices, encouraging regular physical activity, and ensuring adequate sleep.

- **Consultation with healthcare professionals:** Work closely with healthcare professionals, such as pediatricians, dietitians, or naturopathic doctors, to develop an individualized gut-healing protocol tailored to your child's needs and health status.

By implementing these measures and incorporating prebiotics into your child's diet, you can support their digestive health and potentially alleviate symptoms associated with ADHD. However, it is essential to approach these strategies holistically and seek guidance from informed experts to ensure safe and effective implementation.

Tips for Nurturing a Healthy Gut in Children

A healthy digestive tract is like a secret superpower that can empower our kids to thrive in every aspect of their lives. The benefits of caring for it are endless, from boosting immunity to supporting mood and cognitive function.

So, how can we ensure our children's tummies are happy and healthy? Join me as we uncover practical tips and strategies for building a solid foundation of gut health in our young ones. We'll look at the power of gut-friendly foods, the importance of physical activity, and the magic of emotional well-being in nurturing happy bellies and flourishing minds.

This is a journey of love, care, and gut-friendly goodness. Our children's health and happiness await, so here are some strategies to foster a healthy digestive system:

- **Focus on gut-friendly foods:** Ensure your child's diet includes plenty of fiber, prebiotics, and probiotic foods that align with your child's tastes. These nourishing options lay the foundation for a thriving gut microbiome.

- **Promote physical activity:** Encourage regular physical activity while limiting screen time. Exercise aids digestion and promotes better sleep, essential for maintaining gut health.

- **Prioritize emotional well-being:** Dedicate quality family time, practice mindfulness, and foster positive social connections. Emotional well-being is closely linked to gut health, so nurturing positive emotions is critical.

By implementing these tips, you're contributing to a healthy belly in your child and nurturing their overall health and well-being. This holistic approach can bolster their immune system, uplift their mood, and enhance their cognitive abilities.

Gut Feeling: Jake's Journey to Improved Attention Through Healing His Gut-Brain Connection

Jake's exploration of the gut-brain connection and its impact on attention has been enlightening. After being taught about the intricate relationship between his gut health and cognitive function, Jake and his parents took the necessary steps to heal his digestive health for improved attention.

Initially, Jake's diet lacked diversity and was filled with processed foods that disrupted his gut microbiome. However, as he learned about the importance of gut health, he began to make intentional dietary changes. He nurtured a healthier gut environment by incorporating probiotic-rich foods like yogurt, kefir, fermented vegetables, and fiber-rich fruits and vegetables.

As his digestive health improved, Jake noticed significant changes in his attention levels and ability to focus. He experienced fewer distractions and a greater ability to concentrate, improving his performance in various aspects of his life.

Jake's experience underscores the profound impact that healing the gut can have on attention and mental function. Through making beneficial changes to his diet and incorporating gut-healthy foods into his meals, he discovered the power of nutrition in nurturing a healthy gut-brain connection, paving the way for his enhanced attention and overall well-being.

CREATING A POSITIVE MEALTIME ENVIRONMENT

In the cacophony of modern life, amid the plethora of distractions and demands, mealtimes often become a hurried affair, relegated to mere necessity rather than a cherished opportunity for connection and nourishment. Yet for children, the dining table holds a profound significance beyond mere sustenance—it is a place where lifelong habits are formed, relationships are nurtured, and values are instilled.

This chapter delves into creating a positive mealtime environment for kids. It recognizes the pivotal role of this time in shaping children's attitudes toward food and fostering healthy eating behaviors. By implementing strategies such as promoting healthy dietary habits, encouraging mindful eating, and involving children in meal planning and preparation, you can transform shared meals into a joyful and enriching experience that nourishes the body and soul.

In the upcoming sections, you will delve into practical strategies for cultivating healthy eating habits in children. You will also learn how to foster a more profound sense of engagement with food by promoting thoughtful eating practices and actively involving your child in deciding what to eat and making their meals.

Encouraging children to pay attention to their senses and savor each bite cultivates a more conscious approach to eating. At the same time, participation in meal-related activities empowers them to make informed choices about their food. Through these efforts, you can instill lifelong habits prioritizing nutrition and well-being, laying the foundation for a healthy relationship with food that will follow your children as they mature.

Strategies for Fostering Healthy Eating Habits and Positive Behaviors During Meals

In the hustle and bustle of daily life and the challenges of balancing work, school, and other commitments, meals tend to be rushed and chaotic. However, the importance of fostering healthy mealtime habits and positive behaviors while eating cannot be overstated, particularly in shaping children's and adults' nutritional health and overall well-being.

This section explores strategies for creating a nurturing and supportive meal environment where nutritious eating habits are cultivated and positive behaviors are encouraged. These strategies range from building a pleasant and relaxed atmosphere at the dining table to gradually introducing new foods and modeling healthy eating behaviors. Each strategy promotes mindfulness and a positive relationship with food.

Let's explore techniques and tips for healthy eating habits and positive meal behaviors, empowering you and your family to enjoy nourishing and fulfilling eating experiences.

Promoting Positive Mealtime Behaviors

Here are some suggestions you can take to develop healthy habits in children and stimulate positive mealtime behaviors:

Create a Pleasant and Relaxed Eating Environment

- Set the table with colorful and inviting place settings.

- Minimize distractions such as the TV being on or using phones and tablets during meals.

- Encourage pleasant conversation and positive interactions at the table.

Introduce New Foods Gradually

- Offer new foods alongside familiar favorites to reduce resistance.

- Start with small portions of the unfamiliar food and gradually increase exposure to it over time.

- Be patient and persistent, as it may take several attempts for children to accept new foods.

Model Healthy Eating Behaviors

- Serve as a role model by demonstrating enthusiasm for healthy foods.

- Eat meals together as a family whenever possible.

- Enjoy and appreciate various foods, including fruits, vegetables, whole grains, and lean proteins.

Establish Consistent Mealtime Routines

- Set regular meal and snack times to help regulate hunger and prevent grazing.

- Encourage children to take part in meal planning and preparation to nurture a sense of ownership and excitement.

- Stick to a predictable dietary structure, including a balanced combination of protein, carbohydrates, and fats.

Encourage Exploration and Variety

- To expose children to diverse flavors and textures, offer various foods from different food groups.

- Allow kids to explore and experiment with food at their own pace.

- Celebrate small victories and progress, even if it's just trying a bite of a new food.

Make Healthy Eating Fun and Engaging

- Get creative with food presentation by arranging colorful fruits and vegetables in interesting shapes.

- Involve children in gardening or shopping for fresh produce to instill appreciation for wholesome foods.

- Incorporate themed meals or cooking activities to make healthy eating an enjoyable experience.

By employing these approaches, you, as parents and caregivers, can establish a positive meal setting that encourages healthy eating habits and nurtures positive behaviors in your children. Consistency, patience, and creativity are crucial to cultivating a lifelong appreciation for nutritious foods and joyful experiences.

Encouraging Mindful Eating and Avoiding Distractions

It's essential to educate your child about recognizing their physical hunger and fullness cues and encourage them to engage all their senses while eating. This involves minimizing distractions like screens or toys during meals.

You can also introduce simple, practical techniques such as taking small bites, chewing slowly, and savoring the flavors of the food to promote a more conscious and enjoyable experience. By incorporating these practices into their daily routines, your child can better appreciate their consumption.

Encouraging these habits and minimizing distractions is essential for children with ADHD to develop the ability to stay focused. Children can better tune into their hunger and fullness cues when they can concentrate, improving their eating behaviors and overall well-being.

Here are some strategies to promote mindful eating:

- **Create a calm environment:** Minimize distractions such as electronic devices, loud noises, or meal interruptions. Set a calm and peaceful atmosphere to help children focus on their food.

- **Practice mindful eating techniques:** Encourage children to pay attention to their food's taste, texture, and smell. Encourage them to chew slowly and enjoy each bite, fostering a deeper appreciation for the eating experience.

- **Engage the senses:** Guide your child to use their senses to explore their food. Ask them to describe different foods' colors, shapes, and flavors, promoting awareness and engagement with their meals.

- **Offer nutrient-dense foods:** Provide a variety of nutrient-dense foods that nourish the body and support optimal brain function. Include fruits, vegetables, whole grains, lean proteins, and healthy fats in meals and snacks.

- **Practice gratitude:** Encourage children to express gratitude for the food they have and the effort that went into preparing it. Cultivating a sense of thankfulness can enhance the eating experience and promote positive associations with mealtimes.

- **Lead by example:** Children are more likely to adopt healthy habits when they see them practiced by adults, so model mindful eating behaviors by demonstrating attentiveness and appreciation for food.

- **Be patient and supportive:** Understand that learning to eat mindfully takes time, especially for children with ADHD who may struggle with attention and impulsivity. Be patient and offer support and encouragement along the way.

- **Family connection:** Studies have shown several benefits of eating meals together. While it improves family relationships, it also makes kids more likely to explore new foods and develop a better idea of portion control. Statistically, kids who eat with their families have better grades, are happier, and have higher self-esteem and resilience.

Children with ADHD can often struggle with healthy eating habits and food-related behaviors. However, you can be crucial in promoting healthy eating and improving your child's relationship with food. By encouraging behaviors such as slowing down, savoring each bite, and reducing distractions during meals, you can help your child build a positive and sustainable relationship with food. This can lead to improved overall health and well-being.

Involving Children in Meal Planning and Preparation to Increase Their Engagement

Involve your children with ADHD in planning and preparing meals, as this can significantly benefit their overall well-being and development. Parents and caregivers like yourself can enhance children's engagement with food and instill a sense of ownership over their meals by including them in activities such as choosing recipes, grocery shopping, and cooking. This involvement imparts valuable life skills and motivates children to make healthier food choices while fostering a positive relationship with food.

Additionally, participating in meal-related tasks can boost your child's confidence and self-esteem as they see the direct impact of their contributions to the family's meals. Overall, involving kids with ADHD in meal planning and preparation empowers them to participate actively in their dietary habits and promotes a healthier lifestyle. Let us have a look at some examples of the advantages of this practice:

- **Increased engagement with food:** When children with ADHD are engaged in meal planning and preparation, they become more invested in their food choices. Participating in decision-making makes them more likely to try new foods and flavors, leading to a more varied and nutritious diet.

- **Sense of ownership:** Allowing children to have a say in food choices and preparation gives them a sense of ownership over their meals. This can be empowering for those with ADHD, who may struggle with feelings of lack of control in other areas of their lives. Being involved and valued in making decisions can boost their confidence and self-esteem.

- **Development of life skills:** Engaging children in the kitchen helps them develop essential life skills, such as planning, organizing, and following instructions. These skills are particularly beneficial for children with ADHD, as they can improve their executive functioning and ability to focus on tasks.

- **Quality family time:** Meal planning and preparation can provide quality family time and bonding opportunities. Collaborating in the kitchen encourages communication, teamwork, and shared experiences, strengthening family relationships and creating lasting memories.

- **Educational opportunities:** Involving children in meal planning and preparation offers chances for them to learn about nutrition, cooking techniques, and food safety. During this time, you can educate your child about healthy eating habits and the significance of balanced meals.

- **Improving mental health:** Cooking is meditative and creative. It stimulates the senses, and nourishing activities feel good, so it's a win-win!

To make meal planning and preparation a fun and collaborative family activity, consider the following ideas:

- Allow your children to choose a recipe that meets their nutritional guidelines.

- Take your kids grocery shopping and involve them in selecting ingredients, comparing prices, and learning about different food items.

- Assign age-appropriate tasks in the kitchen, such as washing vegetables, stirring ingredients, or setting the table.

- Look for child-friendly recipes that are simple to prepare and allow for creativity, such as homemade pizzas, tacos, or pasta dishes.

- Make meal planning a regular part of your family routine. Involve children in curating a menu and encourage their input.

By involving children with ADHD in meal planning and preparation, you, alongside other parents and caregivers, can promote their engagement with food, foster a sense of ownership, and provide valuable opportunities for learning and bonding as a family.

Cooking Together: Age-Appropriate Kitchen Activities for Kids of All Ages

Incorporating cooking with kids of different ages into your routine is fantastic. Here's how you can integrate age-appropriate cooking activities into a meal plan:

Age-Appropriate Activities

Toddlers (Ages 2–3)

- **Mixing ingredients:** Toddlers can help with simple tasks like mixing ingredients in a bowl. Provide them with a large spoon or spatula and let them stir ingredients together for baking or making simple dishes like salads.

Preschoolers (Ages 4–5)

- **Washing produce:** Under supervision, preschoolers can help wash fruits and vegetables. Teach them about food safety and proper handling techniques while letting them do this important step of meal preparation.

- **Tearing herbs:** Encourage youngsters to help tear herbs or lettuce for salads. This improves their fine motor skills and involves them hands-on in meal preparation.

School-Age Children (Ages 6–10)

- **Cutting soft foods:** Under close supervision, school-age children can start learning basic knife skills by cutting soft foods like bananas, strawberries, or boiled eggs with a child-safe knife.

- **Measuring ingredients:** Teach kids to measure ingredients using measuring cups and spoons. This helps them develop math skills while learning about portion sizes and following recipes.

Preteens and Teens (Ages 11–18)

- **Using the oven:** Older children can safely use the oven under adult supervision. Teach them how to preheat it, use oven mitts, and safely place dishes in and remove them from the oven.

- **Cooking on the stovetop:** Introduce preteens and teens to cooking, starting with simple tasks like stirring and sautéing ingredients. As they gain confidence, they can progress to more advanced techniques like flipping pancakes or scrambling eggs.

Tips for Cooking With Kids

- **Safety first:** Always prioritize safety in the kitchen. Supervise children closely, teach them proper handling techniques, and ensure they use age-appropriate kitchen tools and equipment.

- **Patience and encouragement:** Cooking with kids can be messy and chaotic, but it's also a valuable learning experience. Be patient, offer encouragement, and focus on the fun and educational aspects of creating dishes together.

- **Choose age-appropriate tasks:** Tailor cooking activities to your child's age and skill level. Start with simple tasks and gradually introduce more complex activities as your child gains confidence and proficiency.

- **Make it fun:** Cooking should be enjoyable for kids! Get creative with recipes, involve children in meal planning, and let them express their creativity in the kitchen.

By incorporating cooking activities for your child into meal preparation, you can teach them valuable life skills and foster a love of cooking and healthy eating from a young age.

Dealing With Selective Eaters at Mealtimes

Parents facing the challenge of mealtime with selective eaters often navigate a complex terrain of preferences, aversions, and frustrations. This section offers practical strategies and expert insights to help you transform mealtime struggles into opportunities for growth and connection. From toddlers asserting their independence to teenagers with specific dietary preferences, we address the diverse needs of children at every stage of development.

By understanding the underlying factors contributing to picky eating and implementing tailored approaches, you can encourage healthier eating habits and create a more upbeat dining experience for your entire family. Join us as we empower fellow parents to navigate this path with confidence and compassion.

Suggestions to Improve Mealtimes With a Picky Eater

- **Establish a positive mealtime environment:** Create a relaxed and pleasant atmosphere during meals, free from pressure or coercion. Encourage positive interactions and conversation, making mealtimes an enjoyable experience for everyone.

- **Offer a variety of foods:** Introduce a range of nutritious foods, including fruits, vegetables, whole grains, lean proteins, and dairy products, unless your child has an intolerance or allergen. Encourage exploration and experimentation with different flavors and textures.

- **Boundaries at the dinner table:** Picky eaters can have input, but ultimately, it is your job as a parent to choose the foods on the table. The child decides whether or not to eat them. *Do not* make a separate meal for the picky eater!

- **Involve your child in meal preparation:** Include your child in meal planning, grocery shopping, and cooking activities. This involvement can increase their interest in food and willingness to try new things.

- **Be patient and persistent:** Understand that changing eating behaviors takes time, and progress may be slow. Be patient and continue offering various foods, even if your child initially refuses them.

- **Use positive reinforcement:** Reward your child for trying new foods or exhibiting positive eating behaviors. Offer praise or incentives for adventurous eating, but avoid using food as a bribe or punishment.

- **Set realistic expectations:** Recognize that picky eating is typical for many children and may not necessarily indicate a long-term problem. Focus on gradual progress and celebrate small victories along the way.

- **Seek professional guidance if needed:** If selective eating significantly impacts your child's growth, nutrition, or overall well-being, consult a pediatrician or registered dietitian for personalized advice and support.

Parents often struggle with fussy eaters, but by implementing effective strategies, you can encourage healthy eating habits and improve your children's overall well-being. Creating a positive and enjoyable mealtime experience is critical. It can be achieved by involving children in the kitchen, offering a variety of nutritious foods, and making the dining room a fun and relaxed environment. By following these steps, you can help your picky eaters develop a positive relationship with food that will benefit them throughout their lives.

Streamlining the Eating Process for Picky Eaters

Simplifying the eating process for a picky eater involves implementing strategies to make mealtime less overwhelming and more enjoyable. Here are some ways to accomplish this:

- **Offer familiar foods:** Include familiar and preferred foods in meals to provide comfort and security for the picky eater. Familiarity can help reduce anxiety and resistance to trying new foods.

- **Serve small portions:** Presenting less sizeable portions of food can make a meal more manageable for your child. Start with small servings of new or less preferred foods, gradually increasing the portion size as they become more comfortable.

- **Create a positive environment:** Foster a positive and relaxed atmosphere during mealtimes. Avoid pressuring or coercing your child to eat certain foods, leading to resistance and a negative attitude. Instead, focus on making mealtime enjoyable and stress-free.

- **Offer choices:** Provide the picky eaters options and opportunities to choose what they eat. This can empower them and increase their willingness to try new foods. Offer various nutritious options and let your child decide what to eat.

- **Be patient and persistent:** Changing eating habits takes time. It requires patience and persistence, even if your child is initially hesitant. Continue to provide a variety of foods and gently encourage your picky eater to experiment with new options. Refrain from forcing or pressuring them.

- **Make meals fun:** Include fun and interactive elements with meals. Consider serving foods in interesting shapes or arranging them on colorful plates. Involving a selective eater in meal preparation can make the experience more enjoyable for them.

- **Celebrate progress:** Acknowledge and celebrate small victories and progress made toward expanding your child's food choices. Positive reinforcement can help promote adventurous eating behaviors and encourage continued exploration.

By simplifying the eating process and creating a positive mealtime environment, you can help your child develop healthier eating habits and expand their food preferences over time.

The chapter "Creating a Positive Mealtime Environment" focuses on fostering a supportive and enjoyable atmosphere during meals, particularly for children with fussy eating habits. This underscores the significance of establishing a positive mealtime routine, encouraging open communication, and minimizing stress and pressure surrounding food.

Some key strategies we have introduced include cultivating a relaxed atmosphere, providing a variety of nutritious foods, engaging your child in meal planning and preparation, and celebrating small victories.

By reading this chapter, you have discovered the power of consistency, patience, and encouragement to nurture healthy habits and boost your child's well-being.

Feeding the Soul: Jake's Journey to Enjoying a Nurturing Mealtime Environment

Jake's experience with his parents as they created a positive mealtime environment has been transformative for him and his family. Recognizing the importance of fostering a healthy relationship with food and each other, Jake's parents intentionally endeavored to cultivate a positive atmosphere during meals.

Initially, meals were chaotic. They were filled with distractions and stress, inhibiting the whole family's enjoyment of food and bonding. However, the Thompsons implemented strategies to create a more serene and supportive environment. They set aside dedicated time for eating together, free from distractions like phones or the TV. This allowed them to focus on each other and the food they were sharing. Additionally, they engaged in meaningful conversations, fostering connection and creating cherished memories around the dinner table.

As a result, Jake experienced a shift in his attitude toward eating. He, along with his parents, began to view mealtimes as opportunities for nourishment of both a physical and emotional kind. This positive shift contributed to a healthier relationship with food and improved the overall well-being of the Thompson family.

Jake's experience highlights the importance of creating a positive environment for fostering healthy eating habits and strengthening familial bonds. Through intentional effort and meaningful connections, Jake and his family transformed their mealtime experience into a source of joy and nourishment.

Supplements and Alternative Therapies for ADHD Symptoms

The rise in ADHD prevalence prompts an escalating demand for effective treatments and interventions to alleviate symptoms and enhance the well-being of those affected. While conventional medications and behavioral therapies have traditionally dominated treatment approaches, there's an increasing interest in exploring additional options like supplements and alternative therapies as potential complements.

Supplements such as omega-3 fatty acids, zinc, magnesium, and vitamins B6 and B12 have attracted attention for their potential roles in supporting brain health and addressing ADHD symptoms. These nutrients are thought to play critical roles in neurotransmitter function, cognitive function, and mood regulation, thus serving as potential intervention targets in managing ADHD. Additionally, herbal supplements and botanical extracts like ginkgo biloba and ginseng have been studied for their potential cognitive-enhancing effects and ability to support attention and focus.

In addition to supplements, alternative therapies such as acupuncture, mindfulness meditation, yoga, and neurofeedback are also being explored as potential options for managing ADHD symptoms. These treatments aim to tackle the underlying factors contributing to the condition, such as stress, anxiety, and impaired self-regulation, by promoting relaxation, enhancing attentional control, and refining emotional regulation.

Although the evidence for the effectiveness of these therapies in ADHD management is still emerging, many families are attracted to their holistic and noninvasive nature, as well as their potential to complement traditional remedies.

The growing interest in supplements and alternative therapies reflects a broader shift toward a more integrative and personalized approach to health care, where multiple modalities are considered and combined to tailor treatment to each patient's needs. While further research is necessary to understand the efficacy and safety of these approaches fully, they offer promising avenues for exploring new ways to support children with ADHD on their journey toward improved well-being and functioning.

This chapter examines a variety of supplements and alternative therapies that have been studied for their potential benefits in managing ADHD symptoms. From omega-3 fatty acids and zinc supplements to mindfulness meditation and neurofeedback training, each approach provides a unique perspective on supporting children with this disorder.

Follow along as we explore the research, evidence, and practical considerations surrounding various options for treating ADHD. We aim to empower families like yours to make informed decisions about available options.

Understanding the Role of Supplements in Supporting ADHD Symptoms

Understanding the role of supplements in supporting ADHD symptoms in children is crucial for holistic management. While supplements should not replace prescribed medication or therapy, they can complement traditional treatments and enhance overall well-being. For example, improved attention and cognitive function have been linked to the omega-3 fatty acids found in fish oil.

Nutrients such as zinc, magnesium, and vitamins B6 and B12 also contribute to neurotransmitter function and mood regulation, potentially alleviating hyperactivity and inattention symptoms. However, it's vital to consult healthcare professionals to ensure your child receives safe and appropriate supplementation.

Integrating supplements into a comprehensive treatment plan that includes behavioral therapy, educational support, lifestyle adjustments, and parental education is essential. By combining these strategies, you, as parents and caregivers, can optimize your child's ADHD management and quality of life.

Here's a breakdown of some supplements commonly used for ADHD support:

- **Omega-3 fatty acids:** Omega-3s are known for their brain-boosting benefits. Research suggests that supplementation with these acids may improve attention and behavior and symptoms of sadness and depression in children with ADHD.

- **Zinc:** This mineral is crucial in neurotransmitter function; it may help regulate dopamine levels, which can impact attention and focus.

- **Magnesium:** A deficiency of magnesium has been linked to ADHD symptoms. Aside from addressing this, supplementing with this nutrient may support cognitive function and mood stability.

- **Herbal remedies:** Certain herbs, like ginkgo biloba, ginseng, and passionflower, are sometimes used in alternative medicine for ADHD management. However, evidence supporting their efficacy is limited, and they may interact with other medications or have unpleasant side effects.

- **Iron:** Researchers have found that lacking iron can cause symptoms resembling ADHD. Ensuring adequate intake through supplements or iron-rich foods may benefit children with inattention or excessive movement.

- **Vitamin B6:** Involved in neurotransmitter production, including dopamine and serotonin. Some studies indicate that B6 supplementation may improve ADHD symptoms, especially in children with low levels of this vitamin.

- **Probiotics:** Gut health is linked to brain function, and preliminary research suggests a potential connection between probiotics and ADHD symptoms (Cickovski et al., 2023). Probiotic supplements may indirectly support ADHD management by promoting a healthy gut microbiome. Certain herbs, such as ginkgo biloba, ginseng, and bacopa monnieri, have been researched for their cognitive-enhancing effects. However, further investigation is needed to confirm their effectiveness, particularly for ADHD treatment.

Consulting with your healthcare professional before introducing supplements is vital, as they can interact with medications or have adverse effects on some children. Additionally, supplements should be part of your child's comprehensive treatment plan, complementing behavioral interventions, educational support, and prescribed medications. By adopting a holistic approach to ADHD management incorporating some or all of these elements, you can provide optimal support for your children's overall well-being.

Exploring Holistic and Alternative Therapies to Complement Nutritional Interventions

When addressing ADHD symptoms in children, exploring holistic and alternative therapies alongside nutritional interventions provides a multifaceted approach that acknowledges the interconnectedness of the various factors influencing the condition. By delving into these complementary practices, we, as caregivers, can tap into a broader spectrum of strategies to alleviate our children's symptoms.

This section examines a diverse range of holistic and alternative therapies, each offering unique benefits in supporting children with ADHD. Through this lens, we will navigate the landscape of ADHD management, embracing a holistic understanding that encompasses physical, mental, and emotional dimensions to foster optimal outcomes and enrich the lives of children grappling with ADHD.

From behavioral therapy to mindfulness practices, yoga, and beyond, integrating these approaches into a comprehensive treatment plan underscores the importance of personalized care that is tailored to each child's needs. Here is a brief exploration of each:

- **Behavioral therapy:** Techniques like cognitive-behavioral therapy (CBT) or behavioral parent training help kids develop coping strategies, improve impulse control, and manage symptoms effectively by changing their behavior patterns and thoughts.

- **Mindfulness and meditation:** Meditation changes your brain structure as it thickens the prefrontal cortex, the brain area involved in attention. For your child with ADHD, this can reduce impulsivity, aid stress management, and improve self-regulation and focus.

- **Yoga:** Combining improved physical posture, breathwork, and meditation promotes relaxation, focus, and body awareness. Research indicates that yoga can enhance attention, behavior, and emotional regulation in children diagnosed with ADHD. It also provides a non-competitive environment for children to build their confidence and self-esteem.

- **Acupuncture:** Inserting thin needles into specific points in the body promotes balance and harmony in energy flow, potentially reducing hyperactivity and improving attention.

- **Neurofeedback:** This practice trains participants to regulate their brainwave patterns, which improves attention, impulse control, and executive function by providing real-time feedback on brain activity. While more research is needed, some studies have shown promising results in reducing ADHD symptoms.

- **Aromatherapy:** Essential oils like lavender and peppermint have calming or focusing effects that can complement ADHD management when used cautiously.

- **Music therapy:** Music-based interventions improve attention, self-expression, and emotional regulation, providing a creative outlet for children with ADHD.

- **Regular exercise:** Swimming, running, bicycling, and martial arts are great for kids with ADHD.

- **Dietary modifications:** Some children see relief from their ADHD symptoms when they make dietary changes, such as avoiding or eliminating artificial additives, food colorings, preservatives, gluten, or dairy products. Implementing an elimination diet may help identify specific foods that exacerbate your child's symptoms.

With the success of holistic and alternative therapies as complements to nutritional interventions in managing ADHD, it becomes evident that a multifaceted approach is essential for addressing the complex nature of the condition. By embracing diverse strategies such as behavioral therapy, mindfulness practices, acupuncture, and regular exercise, you can provide comprehensive support that extends beyond symptom management to enhance the overall health of your child with ADHD.

Integrative medicine acknowledges the individuality of each child, recognizing that what works for one may not work for another. Through collaboration among healthcare professionals, educators, parents, and caregivers, we can strive to optimize outcomes and empower children with ADHD to thrive in all aspects of their lives. With continued research, innovation, and a holistic understanding of the condition, we can pave the way for brighter futures and greater possibilities for children navigating the challenges of this neurodevelopmental disorder.

Consulting With Health Care Professionals

Consulting with your child's healthcare professionals is crucial when considering supplements and alternative therapies for managing ADHD symptoms. Professionals such as pediatricians, nutritionists, and naturopaths have the expertise to provide personalized guidance tailored to your child's unique needs. They can perform comprehensive evaluations to pinpoint potential medical conditions or nutritional imbalances that could influence symptoms.

Additionally, these professionals can evaluate potential interactions between supplements and your child's prescribed medications, ensuring that any interventions are safe and appropriate. By collaborating with health experts, you can develop a comprehensive treatment plan that integrates both conventional and alternative approaches, maximizing the effectiveness of ADHD management while prioritizing your child's safety and wellness.

Here's why it is essential to involve healthcare professionals in the holistic treatment process:

- **Individualized assessment:** Professionals can thoroughly assess your child's health history, symptoms, and nutritional status to determine the most appropriate interventions. It is essential to identify any underlying medical conditions or nutritional deficiencies that could be contributing to ADHD symptoms.

- **Medication interactions:** If your child takes any medications for ADHD or other conditions, experts can evaluate potential interactions between supplements and medications. Certain supplements can affect the effectiveness of medications or increase the risk of side effects.

- **Dosage and safety:** Professionals can recommend the appropriate dosage of supplements based on your child's age, weight, and individual needs. They can also ensure that supplements are sourced from reputable manufacturers and are free from contaminants or allergens.

- **Monitoring and follow-up:** They can monitor your child's progress and adjust their treatment plans. Regular appointments allow for ongoing assessment of the effectiveness and safety of supplements and alternative therapies.

- **Educational support:** Experts can provide valuable education and resources to help you make informed decisions about managing your child's symptoms. They can guide you on healthy eating habits, lifestyle modifications, and evidence-based interventions.

- **Holistic approach:** By consulting with a multidisciplinary team of medical professionals, you can take a holistic approach to your child's treatment. This may include integrating nutritional interventions, behavioral therapies, and alternative solutions to address all aspects of your child's well-being.

Remember that every child is unique, and what works for one may not work for another. By collaborating with healthcare professionals, you can develop the best treatment plan that meets your child's needs and maximizes their potential for success.

Embracing a Holistic Approach to Managing Your Child's ADHD Symptoms

Embracing a holistic approach to managing your child's ADHD symptoms requires a comprehensive understanding of their overall well-being. It entails not only addressing the physical manifestations of the condition but also delving into the emotional and cognitive aspects, as well as considering the influence of social interactions and environmental factors. By recognizing and attending to these multifaceted dimensions, parents and caregivers like yourself can create a supportive framework for children's development and success.

This approach integrates various strategies, including optimizing nutrition to support brain function, implementing lifestyle modifications to promote stability and routine, utilizing behavioral interventions to cultivate coping mechanisms and self-regulation, and exploring alternative therapies to complement traditional treatments. Through a balanced approach, you can empower your children to navigate the challenges of ADHD with resilience and confidence, fostering symptom management and overall growth and well-being.

Comprehensive ADHD Management

A comprehensive management strategy for treating ADHD symptoms includes:

- **Medical interventions:** Healthcare professionals may prescribe medications like stimulants (e.g., methylphenidate, amphetamines) or nonstimulants (e.g., atomoxetine, guanfacine) to manage ADHD symptoms. Regular monitoring ensures optimal dosage and effectiveness.

- **Behavioral therapy:** Techniques such as CBT and behavior modification aim to teach coping skills, enhance impulse control, and improve organizational abilities, empowering children to manage their symptoms effectively.

- **Nutritional support:** Collaboration with a nutritionist helps develop a balanced diet rich in omega-3 fatty acids, zinc, magnesium, and vitamins B6 and B12, which are known to support brain function and help manage ADHD symptoms.

- **Lifestyle modifications:** Creating a supportive environment at home and school involves establishing consistent routines, providing organizational tools, promoting regular exercise, ensuring adequate sleep, and minimizing stressors.

- **Educational support:** Collaborating with educators to implement accommodations and modifications in the classroom helps meet your child's unique learning needs, providing additional support and fostering academic success.

- **Emotional connection:** Kids with ADHD are often treated negatively and have three times increased incidence of depression and anxiety and twice the incidence of alcohol misuse, and they start drinking much earlier than their non-ADHD peers (Watson, 2008). Emotional connection gives them a sense of safety, and positive reinforcements make a big difference, even for the most minor actions. Even 10 minutes of one-on-one time with you or your partner, a grandparent, or a sibling can be beneficial.

- **Alternative therapies:** Integrating complementary approaches like mindfulness meditation, yoga, neurofeedback, or music therapy can offer additional support for managing ADHD symptoms.

- **Parental education and support:** Educating yourself about ADHD, training in behavioral management techniques, and offering emotional support are essential for effective caregiving and promoting positive outcomes.

- **Regular monitoring and follow-up:** Ongoing assessment by healthcare professionals ensures the effectiveness and tolerability of interventions, allowing for adjustments to optimize treatment.

- **Consistent routine and structure:** Establishing predictable daily routines and clear expectations helps children feel organized and in control, reducing their anxiety and improving their behavior.

- **Social support:** Encouraging engagement in social activities and fostering positive peer relationships promotes the development of social skills and enhances self-esteem, contributing to overall well-being.

By adopting a holistic approach to managing ADHD, you can address your child's diverse needs and support their journey toward improved happiness. Consulting with healthcare professionals and implementing tailored interventions ensures that each aspect of your child's health is considered, leading to optimal outcomes and a brighter future.

Jake's Journey: Exploring Supplements and Therapies for Managing ADHD Symptoms

Jake's exploration of supplements and alternative therapies for managing his ADHD symptoms has been eye-opening. When they recognized the limitations of traditional treatment approaches, Jake's parents decided to explore complementary methods that could support his overall well-being.

Initially, the Thompsons were skeptical about the effectiveness of these treatment options. However, as they delved deeper into the research and consulted with experts, they discovered many promising options.

From omega-3 fatty acids to zinc and magnesium supplements, Jake found that increasing his intake of certain nutrients could help alleviate his symptoms and improve his cognitive function. Additionally, alternative practices such as mindfulness meditation, neurofeedback, and acupuncture provided him with valuable tools for managing his stress levels and enhancing his focus.

Through trial and error, Jake and his parents identified the best combination of supplements and therapies. Over time, he experienced a noticeable reduction in symptoms, including hyperactivity and inattention, and gained a greater sense of control over his condition.

This experience underscores the importance of a holistic approach to managing ADHD. By exploring supplements and alternative therapies in conjunction with traditional treatments, Jake was able to bolster his treatment plan and achieve significant improvements in his symptoms and overall quality of life.

NAVIGATING SCHOOL AND SOCIAL SITUATIONS

This chapter focuses on fostering a healthy environment for your child at school and during social events. As a parent, you aim for your child to excel academically and in every aspect of life. Essential to this is ensuring they access proper nutrition, navigate school dynamics, and handle peer pressure with resilience and confidence.

Proper nutrition forms the basis of your child's physical health, cognitive development, and emotional well-being. However, ensuring that your child eats well can sometimes pose a challenge amid the daily hustle and bustle. To help you overcome these challenges, this chapter explores strategies for promoting healthy eating habits at school and during social gatherings. From packing nutritious lunches to advocating for better cafeteria options, you'll explore practical ways to ensure your child with ADHD receives the nourishment they need to excel in and out of the classroom.

Establishing effective communication with teachers and school administration is crucial in creating a supportive educational environment for your child. Clear and respectful conversations are essential when addressing dietary concerns, advocating for your child's needs, or learning about school policies. Let's establish positive relationships with school staff, effectively conveying concerns and collaborating toward solutions that benefit your child's overall well-being and academic success.

Navigating the social landscape of school can be exciting and daunting for children. Peer pressure, social dynamics, and the desire to fit in can present challenges that require parental guidance and support. This chapter, therefore, explores strategies for helping your child develop resilience, assertiveness, and confidence in the face of peer pressure. From teaching them to make healthy choices independently to providing tools for asserting boundaries respectfully, you and your child will be empowered to navigate school and social situations gracefully and confidently.

Now that you know what to expect, you can start cultivating a supportive atmosphere where your child can thrive academically, emotionally, and socially. Once you're equipped with the relevant knowledge and strategies, you'll be able to promote proper nutrition, foster effective communication, and empower your child to navigate the complexities of school and their social life with resilience and confidence.

Tips for Promoting Proper Nutrition at School and During Social Events

Parenting a child with ADHD presents distinctive challenges, particularly in ensuring they uphold a balanced diet while at school or participating in social gatherings. As soon as you're armed with the practical guidance and strategies this section presents, you can assist your child in making nutritious food choices, whether in the cafeteria or at a get-together with friends.

We will start by discussing tips for packing healthy lunches and snacks. Then, we will explore navigating school cafeteria options and managing the challenges of social events and parties. Ensuring your child maintains a nutritious diet may require additional effort and preparation. Still, the benefits for their overall health and well-being make it worthwhile.

Implementing these tips and strategies for nutritious meals, cafeteria choices, and social-event challenges can help your child develop lasting healthy eating habits. Because of this lifelong impact, it is essential to maintain patience and remain supportive as your child learns to make healthier choices. Remember also to celebrate their successes along the way.

Packing Healthy Lunches and Snacks

It is vital to provide a child with ADHD with a healthy, balanced schooltime meal to help fuel their brain and maintain focus in the classroom. A nutritious lunch and snacks can provide the necessary nutrients to keep them energized and alert throughout the school day. Additionally, sending them to school with a packed lunch means that your child is relying on something other than unhealthy cafeteria options for sustenance. With some planning, you can prepare your child for academic success and a healthier lifestyle. Here are some tips to consider:

- **Plan ahead:** Set aside time weekly to plan your child's lunches and snacks. Involve them to increase their buy-in and make them more likely to eat what you pack.

- **Include a variety of foods:** In every meal, try to include different options from all the food groups. Add fruits, vegetables, whole grains, lean proteins, and healthy fats. This ensures that your child has a balanced diet that provides sustained energy throughout the day.

- **Focus on finger foods:** Foods that are easy to eat by hand are often more appealing to children with ADHD. Think carrot sticks, cherry tomatoes, grapes, and whole grain crackers.

- **Prep in advance:** Simplify busy mornings by prepping fruits, veggies, and snacks over the weekend for quick and easy access when filling your child's lunchbox.

- **Limit sugary treats:** While an occasional treat is fine, limit the number of sugary snacks and drinks in your child's lunchbox. These foods can lead to energy crashes and difficulty focusing later in the day.

Navigating School Cafeteria Options

School cafeterias can be overwhelming environments for children with ADHD, given the multitude of food choices and distractions. The bustling atmosphere, crowded tables, and sensory stimuli can easily overload their senses and impede their ability to focus on eating or socializing.

Additionally, the absence of structure and routine in cafeteria settings can worsen impulsivity and distractibility, posing challenges for children with ADHD to make healthy food choices and participate suitably in social interactions. You and your educators can support your child by guiding them in navigating this environment. You can do this by creating visual schedules for them, practicing mindfulness techniques at home, and encouraging healthy eating habits.

Advocating for quieter, less stimulating lunch spaces or designated quiet zones can help minimize distractions and promote a more conducive experience for children with ADHD. Addressing these challenges proactively, you can help your child with ADHD better navigate cafeterias and enjoy more positive lunchtime experiences.

Here's how you can help your child navigate choices of what to eat:

- **Review the cafeteria menu together:** Take some time to review the school menu with your child each week. Discuss the healthiest options and encourage them to make informed choices.

- **Encourage balance:** Teach your child to create balanced meals by choosing foods from different groups. Encourage them to include fruits, vegetables, and whole grains whenever possible.

- **Pack a backup:** If your child needs clarification about the cafeteria options or tends to make impulsive choices, consider packing a backup lunch or snacks they can rely on.

- **Advocate for healthier options:** If the school cafeteria lacks healthy choices, consider speaking to the school's administration team about introducing better options or providing nutrition education for students.

- **Communication:** Initiate open communication with the administrators, teachers, or cafeteria staff to collaborate on promoting healthy food choices for your child during school hours.

Managing the Challenges of Social Events and Parties

Social events and parties pose unique challenges for children with ADHD, particularly when it comes to navigating decisions about what to eat. The excitement, noise, and sensory overload common at these gatherings can overwhelm affected children, making it difficult for them to regulate their behavior and make healthy food choices. Furthermore, the abundance of sugary snacks, fast food, and treats that are often available at such events can exacerbate hyperactivity and impulsivity in children with the condition.

You and other parents and caregivers can support your children by planning and offering nutritious alternatives, such as fruit platters, veggie trays, and protein-rich snacks. Providing clear expectations, setting boundaries around food choices, and offering guidance on portion control and mindful eating can also help children with ADHD make healthier choices at social events. Empowering them with the necessary tools and support allows them to successfully navigate social situations and enjoy positive experiences at parties and gatherings.

Here's how you can help your child navigate these situations:

- **Communicate with hosts:** If your child is attending a party or social event, consider contacting the host in advance to discuss any dietary restrictions or preferences. To minimize inconvenience, offer to bring a dish your child enjoys that fits their nutritional needs.

- **Provide guidance:** Before the event, talk to your child about how they can make good choices while still enjoying themselves. Before they indulge in treats, encourage them to have healthier options like fruits and vegetables first.

- **Offer support:** If your child feels overwhelmed or unsure about what to eat at a social event, offer them support and guidance. Help them navigate the food options and make choices that align with their dietary goals.

- **Lead by example:** Be a role model for your child by making better food choices yourself. Show them that nutritious eating is important for everyone, not just those with ADHD.

Communicating With Teachers and School Administration

Clear and open communication with teachers and school administrators is crucial when advocating for a child with ADHD. It guarantees that kids receive the essential support and accommodations to excel academically and socially. Encouraging open and collaborative dialogue allows you to offer valuable insights into your child's strengths, challenges, and specific needs related to their ADHD. This includes sharing information about effective strategies, preferred learning styles, and any accommodations or modifications that have been beneficial in the past.

Additionally, you can work with educators to develop personalized education plans (IEPs), or 504 plans, that outline specific accommodations, such as extended time on assignments, preferential seating, or behavioral interventions, to support your child's academic success. Regular communication and ongoing collaboration between you and school staff are essential to monitor progress, address concerns, and ensure a supportive learning environment that meets your child's needs.

Here are some tips for effective communication:

- **Initiate open communication:** Reach out to your child's teacher and school administration at the beginning of the school year or as soon as ADHD is diagnosed. Share information about your child's diagnosis, strengths, challenges, and any strategies or accommodations you are trying or have been effective in the past.

- **Establish regular communication channels:** Set up regular meetings or check-ins with your child's teacher to discuss their progress, challenges, and any changes in their needs. This could be through in-person meetings, phone calls, emails, or a communication app used by the school.

- **Provide relevant information:** Share pertinent information about your child's ADHD diagnosis, including any documentation from health care professionals, IEPs, or 504 plans. Educate teachers and school staff about ADHD and its impact on your child's learning and behavior—this can also benefit other affected children.

- **Collaborate on accommodations:** Work with teachers and school staff to develop and implement appropriate accommodations and support systems for your child. This may include seating arrangements, extended time on assignments or tests, preferential seating, frequent breaks, or access to assistive technology.

- **Share strategies for success:** Share strategies that effectively manage your child's ADHD symptoms at home or in other settings. This could include behavior-management techniques, organization strategies, or sensory accommodations that help your child stay focused and engaged.

- **Monitor progress:** Regularly track your child's progress in school and promptly communicate any concerns or changes in their needs to teachers and school administration. Take a proactive approach to addressing issues and work with the relevant school staff to find effective solutions.

- **Be an advocate for your child:** Advocate for your child's needs and rights within the school system. If you encounter resistance or barriers to implementing accommodations, work with school staff to find alternative solutions or seek support from special education services or advocacy organizations.

- **Maintain a positive relationship:** Keep lines of communication open and maintain a positive relationship with teachers and school administration, even if challenges arise. Recognize and appreciate their efforts to support your child and work collaboratively to address any issues that may occur.

By effectively communicating with teachers and school administration, you can ensure that your child receives the support and accommodations they need to thrive in the school environment despite their ADHD diagnosis. Collaboration and teamwork between home and school are essential for your child's success.

Understanding the Importance of Open Communication

Ensuring your child receives the necessary support involves a collaborative effort between you as a parent and the school staff. Central to this partnership is open communication, which serves as the cornerstone for sharing crucial information, insights, and strategies.

Fostering an environment of transparency and mutual understanding, you and educators can effectively address your child's diverse needs. This collaborative approach enhances the effectiveness of interventions and promotes a supportive learning environment where your child can thrive academically, socially, and emotionally.

Sharing Information About Dietary Needs

Dietary habits can significantly impact your child's behavior and cognitive function. As a parent, effectively communicating your child's nutritional needs to teachers and administrators can play a pivotal role in promoting a healthy eating routine. An excellent place for you to start would be by providing comprehensive information about any food sensitivities, allergies, or dietary restrictions your child may have. You can then collaborate with school staff to develop a plan to accommodate your child's needs at school.

Here are some tips for effective communication regarding your child's dietary needs:

- Arrange a dedicated meeting with your child's teachers and relevant school personnel to discuss dietary concerns comprehensively. Ensure this discussion provides ample time to address your child's nutritional requirements and preferences.

- Prepare written documentation detailing your child's specific needs, including preferred snacks and foods to be avoided. This is a valuable reference for school staff and helps ensure consistency in meeting your child's dietary requirements.

- Stress the significance of consistently adhering to nutritional guidelines to support your child's overall well-being and academic performance. Highlighting the direct link between proper nutrition, behavior, and cognitive function can underscore the importance of compliance.

- Foster an atmosphere of open dialogue during your initial meeting, encouraging school staff to share their insights and perspectives on implementing your child's dietary strategies and the relation these measures have to the classroom setting. Inviting feedback promotes collaboration and ensures the nutrition plan is feasible and practical.

Coordinating Strategies for Promoting a Healthy Eating Routine

In addition to sharing information about dietary needs, collaborating with school staff to implement strategies for promoting a healthy eating routine can further support your child's cognitive function and overall health. Work together to establish mealtime routines, incorporate nutritious snacks into the school day, and create a supportive environment that encourages healthy food choices.

Strategies for Promoting Healthy Eating

- Collaborate with administrators to ensure the school offers nutritious meal options in the cafeteria and vending machines.

- Guide your child's teachers on incorporating brain-boosting foods and snacks into classroom activities.

- Advocate for regular breaks and opportunities for physical activity to support overall well-being and appetite regulation in all children.

- Encourage educators to provide positive reinforcement and praise for healthy eating habits to foster a good relationship with food within the school setting.

Fostering Strong Relationships With School Staff

As a parent, it is essential to consider your child's dietary needs, overall well-being, and academic success. Establishing a trusting and healthy relationship with the school's staff is critical to doing this. Open communication and mutual respect help cultivate an environment where effective collaboration and advocacy for your child's success can thrive. This will help ensure your child receives the support they need to achieve their full potential in a safe and nurturing school environment.

Establishing Open Lines of Communication

Initiate regular communication with teachers and school administrators to stay informed about your child's progress, challenges, and emerging needs. Keep channels of communication open for sharing updates, concerns, and insights that can contribute to a comprehensive understanding of your child's strengths and areas for growth.

Fostering effective communication can be managed by implementing specific tips:

- Schedule regular check-ins with teachers via email, phone calls, or in-person meetings to discuss your child's academic and social development.

- Actively listen to the viewpoints and insights of school staff, acknowledging their expertise and contributions to your child's education.

- Provide updates on any changes in your child's routine, medication, or external factors that may impact their behavior or performance at school.

- Collaborate on setting realistic goals and strategies for addressing challenges while leveraging your collective expertise and that of the school staff.

Building a Supportive Partnership

Cultivating a collaborative and supportive partnership with school staff is essential for the academic and social success of children with ADHD. You can foster positive relationships with teachers, counselors, and administrators by demonstrating a willingness to work together toward shared goals and outcomes. This collaborative approach involves open communication, active listening, and mutual respect for expertise and perspectives.

You can show appreciation for the efforts and contributions of school staff by acknowledging their dedication and commitment to supporting the growth and development of all students, including others like your child with ADHD. By working as a team, you and educators can develop effective strategies, implement appropriate accommodations, and provide consistent support to help your child and other children with ADHD thrive while they learn. This partnership promotes a supportive environment that meets the diverse needs of all students and enhances the overall educational experience.

There are several relationship-building strategies to try:

- Attend parent-teacher conferences, school events, and workshops to connect with school staff and demonstrate your commitment to your child's education.

- Volunteer to assist with classroom activities, events, or initiatives to foster a positive rapport with teachers and administrators.

- Advocate for resources, accommodations, and support services to enhance your child's learning experience and promote inclusivity within the school community.

- Express gratitude for the dedication and care demonstrated by school staff in supporting your child's unique needs and journey toward success.

Open communication serves as a powerful catalyst for collaboration, understanding, and advocacy when supporting a child with ADHD. By fostering a culture of transparency, respect, and partnership between yourself, other parents, and school staff, you can create an environment where your child feels valued, supported, and empowered to thrive.

Embrace the opportunity to engage in meaningful dialogue, share insights, and work together with others toward a shared vision of success for all of our children. With the educational figures mentioned in this section, you can nurture your child's true potential and pave the way for a brighter future.

Jake's Triumph: Navigating School and Social Settings With ADHD

Despite facing unique challenges, Jake has learned to adapt and thrive in various environments. His journey in navigating school and social situations with ADHD has been a testament to his resilience and determination, as well as the dedication of his parents.

Jake initially struggled with staying focused and organized in school, which affected his academic performance and confidence. However, with support from his teachers, parents, and healthcare team, he developed strategies to manage his ADHD symptoms effectively. By implementing techniques such as breaking tasks into smaller, more manageable steps, using visual aids, and practicing mindfulness, he improved his concentration and academic outcomes.

Moreover, his challenges extended beyond the classroom and into social situations. Due to his impulsivity and difficulty regulating his emotions, he struggled to maintain friendships and navigate social interactions. Through regular therapy and by attending support groups, he learned valuable social skills and coping mechanisms, enabling him to foster meaningful relationships and navigate social situations with greater confidence and ease.

Jake's experience highlights the importance of understanding and addressing the unique challenges faced by individuals with ADHD in school and social settings. Through perseverance, support, and a willingness to learn and adapt, Jake has overcome obstacles and forged a path toward success and fulfillment in both academic and social spheres.

LIFESTYLE FACTORS FOR OPTIMAL BRAIN HEALTH

This chapter explores simple lifestyle changes that greatly affect your child's cognitive function, focus, and self-control. It will help you further support your child with ADHD. First, we will touch on how regular physical activity benefits the body and the brain. We will start by discussing some good old-fashioned exercise, noting how simple movements can help your child concentrate better and feel calmer.

Next, we will discuss sleep and how getting enough rest is crucial for kids with ADHD. In this exploration, you will discover practical strategies for establishing a better bedtime routine and optimizing your child's sleep environment to ensure they wake up refreshed and prepared to concentrate.

Lastly, we will tackle stress, as this can make ADHD symptoms worse. By creating a calm and supportive atmosphere, you can help your child thrive. To help you do this, we will show you how to reduce your tension levels with relaxation techniques and mindfulness exercises.

Remember, even small changes can significantly improve your child's life. Focusing on exercise, sleep, and stress reduction gives your child the best chance at a healthy and happy life. So, without further ado, let's get started!

The Importance of Regular Exercise, Adequate Sleep, and Stress Reduction

Integrating consistent physical activity, ensuring sufficient sleep, and employing stress-relief methods can significantly help manage your child's ADHD symptoms. By addressing these key lifestyle factors, you can help support their cognitive functioning, emotional regulation, and overall quality of life.

Exercise

While your kid might instead want to be playing PlayStation 5, the reality is that regular movement is immensely beneficial for children with ADHD and a much better use of their time. Some of the benefits of exercise include that it:

- **Boosts brain function:** Physical activity helps to increase blood flow to the brain, enhancing cognitive function and focus, which can be particularly beneficial for kids with ADHD, who may struggle with attention and concentration.

- **Regulates energy levels:** Exercise helps regulate energy levels and improves sleep patterns, which can be erratic in children with ADHD. Better sleep leads to improved attention and behavior during the day.

- **Reduces hyperactivity and impulsivity:** Consistent physical activity is instrumental in mitigating hyperactive and impulsive behaviors often linked to ADHD. It serves as a constructive outlet for surplus energy while aiding your child in developing impulse-management skills.

- **Enhances mood and self-esteem:** Exercise releases endorphins, the "feel-good" chemicals in the brain, which can ease anxiety and depression. Mastering physical skills and participating in sports also boosts self-esteem and confidence.

- **Promotes social interaction:** Engaging in team sports or group activities offers valuable opportunities for social interaction, aiding your child in honing essential social skills such as cooperation, communication, and teamwork.

Incorporating regular exercise into the routine of children with ADHD can significantly enhance their physical health, mental well-being, and overall quality of life. Moreover, it provides a delightful avenue for your child to stay active and engaged while fostering a positive outlook on life.

Adequate Sleep

Getting adequate sleep is crucial for children with ADHD for several reasons, such as:

- **Improved attention and focus:** Sufficient sleep helps regulate attention and concentration, often impaired in children with ADHD. Lack of sleep can exacerbate attention deficits, making it harder for your child to focus on tasks or follow instructions.

- **Emotional regulation:** Sleep plays a vital role in emotional regulation. Children with ADHD often struggle with impulsivity and mood swings, and getting enough sleep helps them stabilize their emotions, reducing the likelihood of meltdowns or outbursts.

- **Behavioral control:** Quality sleep contributes to better behavioral control. Children with ADHD may exhibit impulsive or hyperactive behavior, which is exacerbated by sleep deprivation. Getting enough rest can help mitigate these effects.

- **Memory and learning:** Sleep is pivotal in memory consolidation and learning facilitation. Children with ADHD already grapple with challenges in these areas, and insufficient sleep can worsen difficulties in retaining information and academic performance.

- **Physical health:** Consistent lack of sleep can compromise the immune system, rendering children more vulnerable to illnesses. Prioritizing rest helps support their overall physical health and well-being.

- **Better medication effectiveness:** Many children with ADHD are prescribed medication to manage their symptoms. However, poor sleep habits can compromise the efficacy of these medications. Alternatively, stimulant ADHD medications can interfere with sleep. Ensuring proper rest can optimize the benefits of your child's treatment strategy.

Establishing consistent evening routines and ensuring that your child gets enough rest each night can significantly improve their daily functioning, academic performance, and overall quality of life.

Managing Stress

Reducing the amount of stress on children with ADHD is crucial for several reasons:

- **Reducing overwhelm:** Children with ADHD often experience heightened sensitivity to stressors due to their neurological differences. Stress can exacerbate their symptoms, making it harder for them to focus, regulate their emotions, and control their impulses. Effective management techniques help reduce overwhelm and make it easier for them to navigate daily challenges.

- **Improving attention and focus:** Stress can significantly impair attention and focus in children with ADHD. They can better regulate their attention and concentration levels by managing pressure effectively, improving academic performance and task engagement.

- **Enhancing emotional regulation:** Children with ADHD may struggle with emotional regulation, so they experience intense emotions more frequently than their peers. Techniques like deep breathing exercises and mindfulness practices enable them to cultivate coping mechanisms for regulating emotions and responding to situations more calmly.

- **Promoting social skills:** Stress can interfere with social interactions and relationships, which are already challenging areas for many children with ADHD. Teaching stress management techniques can empower them to handle social situations more effectively, reducing conflicts and enhancing their ability to connect with others.

- **Preventing health issues:** Chronic stress can have detrimental effects on physical health, causing weakened immune function, disrupted sleep patterns, and increased risk of developing anxiety or depression. By learning how to manage pressure early on, children with ADHD can lower their risk of experiencing these health issues later in life.

- **Boosting self-esteem:** Persistent stress can undermine a child's confidence and self-esteem. By teaching them skills to manage this and providing support, you, other caregivers, and educators can help your child with ADHD feel more capable and confident in their abilities to handle challenges effectively.

Ultimately, prioritizing stress management empowers parents and caregivers like you, as well as educators, to foster a supportive environment where children with ADHD can excel academically, socially, and emotionally.

Strategies for Incorporating Physical Activity Into Daily Routines

Integrating physical activity into your child's daily schedule, especially if they have ADHD, can significantly enhance their overall well-being. Here are practical tips to make exercise enjoyable and to seamlessly integrate it into their routine:

- **Schedule regular exercise time:** Allocate dedicated times daily for physical activity, establishing it as a consistent routine.

- **Choose activities they enjoy:** To keep your child motivated, find activities they love, such as team sports, biking, dancing, or swimming.

- **Break it into manageable chunks:** Also known as "exercise snacks," divide activities into smaller sessions throughout the day to accommodate their attention span.

- **Make it fun:** Incorporate games or challenges to make activities engaging, encouraging your child's active participation.

- **Include variety:** Rotate between activities to prevent boredom and stimulate different muscle groups.

- **Encourage outdoor play:** Take advantage of parks and playgrounds for outdoor activities, allowing your child to benefit from nature's therapeutic effects.

- **Be a role model:** Lead by example and engage in physical activities yourself, involving your child whenever possible.

- **Use positive reinforcement:** Offer praise and encouragement to motivate your child's participation in physical activities.

- **Consider structured activities:** Enroll them in programs like team sports or dance classes for social interaction and skill development.

- **Be flexible:** Adapt plans as needed and prioritize consistency over perfection, helping your child recognize that some days may be more challenging.

- **Monitor progress:** Track your child's participation and observe changes in their behavior or mood to tailor activities to their needs.

Remember, making physical activity enjoyable and rewarding fosters a lifelong habit of staying active and healthy for children with ADHD.

Now, it is time for us to explore different exercise and activity options for your child. Here are some suggestions that can be beneficial for a child who struggles with hyperactivity:

Team Sports

- **Soccer:** Involves constant movement and quick decision-making, which can help improve focus and coordination.

- **Basketball:** Fast-paced and requires teamwork, which can help improve social skills and concentration.

- **Volleyball:** Focuses on timing and coordination while also promoting teamwork and communication.

Martial Arts

- **Taekwondo:** Helps with discipline, self-control, and positively channeling energy.

- **Judo:** Teaches control and balance, which can be beneficial for children with ADHD.

- **Karate:** Emphasizes focus, respect, and self-discipline while providing a structured environment.

Yoga and Mindfulness

- **Yoga:** Involves gentle stretching and breathing exercises, which can promote relaxation and improve attention span.

- **Tai chi:** Introduces slow, deliberate movements that can help improve concentration and reduce hyperactivity.

- **Mindfulness meditation:** Teaches children to be present in the moment and manage their emotions effectively.

Individual Sports

- **Swimming:** Provides a full-body workout while soothing and calming for children with ADHD.

- **Cycling:** Helps burn off excess energy while also improving balance and coordination.

- **Gymnastics:** Requires focus, strength, and flexibility, which can benefit children with an attention deficit.

Outdoor Activities

- **Hiking:** Allows children to explore nature while engaging in physical activity and reducing stress.

- **Rock climbing:** Builds strength, problem-solving skills, and confidence in a structured environment.

- **Kayaking or canoeing:** Provides a sense of adventure while improving coordination and focus.

Dance Classes

- **Ballet:** Teaches discipline, grace, and body awareness while improving balance and flexibility.

- **Hip-hop:** Because it is fast-paced and expressive, hip-hop can be a great outlet for children with ADHD to channel their energy.

- **Jazz or modern dance:** Promotes creativity and self-expression while improving coordination and motor skills.

Playground Games

- **Tag or capture the flag:** Promotes running, chasing, and strategic thinking in a fun and social setting.

- **Jump rope:** Improves coordination, rhythm, and cardiovascular fitness playfully.

- **Obstacle courses:** Engage children in physical challenges while stimulating their problem-solving skills.

Remember to choose activities that your child enjoys and feels comfortable with.

Exploring Relaxation Techniques and Mindfulness Practices for ADHD Kids

Helping your child learn about and find relaxation and mindfulness practices that genuinely resonate with them is one of the best things you can do for them. Teaching them about these practices and techniques from a young age is important for several reasons.

First, mindfulness and relaxation can help them manage their emotions and stress better. Children with ADHD often have big feelings and can feel overwhelmed quickly, so mindfulness practices will help them stay calm and centered. It's like giving them a superpower for handling life's ups and downs.

Learning relaxation techniques early on also prepares them for success later in life. It gives them tools to cope with life's challenges, focus better, and even improve their sleep. If you need more incentive, imagine your child being able to tackle homework or handle a challenging situation easily because they've learned how to center themselves. Equipping them with these skills is like giving them their secret weapon against stress.

Let's also remember to build their confidence and self-awareness. When children with ADHD learn to recognize their emotions and how to calm themselves down, they become more in tune with themselves. This self-awareness is priceless and can help them navigate social situations, build better relationships, and feel more comfortable in their skin. Teaching relaxation and mindfulness to your child with ADHD is like giving them a toolbox complete with awesome skills for life. It's a gift that keeps on giving.

Here are some techniques and practices that you can encourage your child to explore:

- **Deep breathing exercises:** Teach your child simple deep breathing techniques. For instance, a simple exercise involves inhaling slowly through the nose for a count of four, holding for the same count, and then exhaling slowly through the mouth for another four counts. Ask your child to repeat this several times.

- **Progressive muscle relaxation:** Guide your child through tensing and relaxing different muscle groups. This can help them become more aware of the tension and learn to release it.

- **Guided imagery:** Use guided imagery scripts or recordings to lead your child through calming visualizations. Encourage them to imagine a peaceful place where they feel safe and relaxed.

- **Mindful walking:** Take mindful walks together, encouraging your child to pay attention to the sensations of each step they take, the sounds around them, and the movement of their body.

- **Body scan meditation:** Guide your child through a body scan meditation, where they focus on each part of their body sequentially, noticing any sensations without judgment.

- **Yoga and stretching:** Practice simple yoga poses or stretching exercises with your child. These can help them release physical tension, and the practices promote relaxation.

- **Mindful eating:** Motivate your child to practice mindful eating by encouraging them to focus on the colors, textures, flavors, and aromas of their food with every bite.

- **Sensory activities:** Entertain your child with sensory activities like playing with kinetic sand, using stress balls, or listening to calming music with headphones.

- **Journaling:** Encourage your child to keep a journal to express their thoughts and feelings. This can help them process their emotions and gain clarity.

- **Mindfulness apps and games:** Explore mindfulness apps and games designed for children. They often include guided meditations, breathing exercises, and relaxation activities in a fun and engaging format.

Remember to approach these practices with patience and understanding and tailor them to suit your child's preferences and needs. It's also a good idea to involve them in determining which techniques they find most helpful.

Introducing and Incorporating These Practices Into Your Child's Daily Routine

Introducing relaxation and mindfulness practices into your child's daily routine can benefit their overall well-being and you as a parent. Here's a simple guide to help you incorporate these practices:

- **Understand the basics:** Ensure you grasp the fundamentals of relaxation and mindfulness before introducing them to your child. This aids in effective explanation.

- **Choose appropriate activities:** Tailor activities to your child's age and interests. For younger children, consider coloring, simple breathing exercises, or storytelling; for older ones, guided meditations, yoga, or nature walks may be preferable.

- **Set a regular schedule:** Establish a consistent daily time slot for relaxation and mindfulness, integrating them into your child's routine—morning, after school, or before bedtime are ideal options.

- **Lead by example:** Model relaxation and mindfulness practices in your routine to encourage your child to follow suit.

- **Start with short sessions:** Begin with brief sessions to prevent overwhelming your child; gradually extend durations as they grow more comfortable with the chosen practices.

- **Create a relaxing environment:** Select a quiet, comfortable space without distractions and consider incorporating dim lighting, soft music, or calming scents like lavender.

- **Teach breathing exercises:** Introduce fundamental breathing techniques such as belly breathing or counting breaths to help your child relax and focus.

- **Practice mindful activities:** Encourage mindful engagement in everyday activities like eating, walking, or playing, emphasizing presence in the moment.

- **Use guided imagery:** Guide your child through relaxing visualizations or imagery exercises, prompting them to vividly imagine peaceful scenes or favorite activities.

- **Be patient and supportive:** Recognize that learning to relax and be mindful requires time and practice. Your child will benefit from you offering patience, encouragement, and support.

- **Celebrate progress:** Acknowledge and celebrate your child's efforts and advancements in integrating these practices. Doing this may nurture their motivation to continue their mindfulness journey.

By following these steps and making relaxation and mindfulness a regular part of your child's routine, you can help them develop valuable stress-management skills, improve their focus, and promote their overall well-being.

Elevating Brain Health: Jake's Journey Through Lifestyle Optimization

Lifestyle factors are crucial in optimizing brain health, and Jake's journey exemplifies the tremendous impact of prioritizing these elements. Jake has unlocked the keys to maintaining optimal brain function and overall well-being with his parents' encouragement and by adopting a holistic approach that encompasses nutrition, exercise, sleep, stress management, and social connections.

His commitment to a balanced diet rich in essential nutrients and regular physical activity has provided his brain with the fuel and stimulation it needs to thrive. Additionally, prioritizing adequate sleep has allowed Jake's brain to recharge and consolidate memories, enhancing his cognitive function and mood regulation.

Moreover, Jake's proactive approach to managing stress through mindfulness practices and cultivating meaningful social connections has further bolstered his mental health. Jake has created an environment conducive to cognitive resilience and emotional well-being by reducing chronic stress and fostering a supportive social network.

Jake's experience underscores the profound impact of lifestyle factors on brain health and highlights the importance of incorporating these practices into daily life for optimal cognitive function and overall vitality.

CONCLUSION

In this book, *Nutrition for ADHD Kids*, you have explored practical strategies for managing ADHD symptoms through nutrition and lifestyle interventions. Each chapter has focused on key concepts and solutions to help reinforce the information provided and empower you to effectively support your child's well-being. You have learned to:

- **Assess current dietary habits:** Take note of what your child eats and identify areas for improvement.

- **Plan balanced meals and snacks:** Use the principles of a balanced diet to ensure your child receives all the essential nutrients.

- **Establish a consistent meal schedule:** Set regular times for breakfast, lunch, dinner, and snacks to regulate appetite and energy levels.

- **Involve your child in meal preparation:** Encourage participation to increase interest in trying new foods and develop essential skills.

- **Offer variety and be patient:** Provide diverse foods and be flexible as your child adjusts to new tastes and textures.

- **Set realistic goals:** Start with small changes and celebrate successes.

- **Monitor progress and stay informed:** Track your child's response to dietary changes and remain updated on nutrition research and recommendations for ADHD.

Following these steps will help you begin implementing improved daily nutrition practices for your child and support their overall well-being.

Parenting Tips for ADHD: Do's and Don'ts

Parenting a child with ADHD comes with unique challenges, but with patience, understanding, and practical strategies such as those contained in this book, supporting your child's well-being and success is possible. You can create a supportive environment that fosters growth and development by educating yourself about the disorder, seeking support from professionals and support groups, and developing tailored strategies to manage your child's symptoms.

Maintaining open communication with your child, providing consistent structure and routines, and celebrating their strengths and accomplishments is crucial. As you do all this, remember to prioritize self-care for yourself as well, as parenting a child with ADHD can be demanding. You can help your child thrive and reach their full potential with love, patience, and perseverance. To better support you in this endeavor, here are some do's and don'ts for parenting a child with ADHD:

What You Should Do

- **Educate yourself:** Learn as much as possible about ADHD, including its symptoms, challenges, and treatment options. Understanding your child's condition will help you better support them and advocate for their needs.

- **Establish routines:** Create consistent routines and schedules for daily activities, including meals, homework, and bedtime. Predictability and structure can help children with attention deficits feel more organized and less overwhelmed.

- **Set clear expectations:** Communicate expectations and rules to your child using straightforward language and visual aids, if necessary. Specify which behaviors are acceptable and outline the consequences for breaking the rules.

- **Encourage positive reinforcement:** Reward your child for their efforts and accomplishments, no matter how small they may be. Positive reinforcement can motivate them to stay focused and engaged in tasks.

- **Break tasks into manageable steps:** Break activities into smaller, more manageable steps to assist your child in staying on track and preventing feelings of being overwhelmed. Provide support and encouragement as they work through each step.

- **Promote physical activity:** Regular physical activity and exercise can help reduce hyperactivity and enhance focus and attention. Find activities that your child enjoys and make them a regular part of their routine.

What You Should Not Do

- **Focus solely on negative behaviors:** Avoid dwelling on your child's mistakes or negative behaviors. Instead, focus on their strengths and efforts and offer constructive feedback and support to help them improve.

- **Use punishment as a primary discipline strategy:** While consequences are essential for shaping behavior, relying solely on punishment can be counterproductive and may damage your relationship with your child. Instead, focus on positive reinforcement and teaching them problem-solving skills.

- **Comparisons:** Avoid comparing your child to their siblings or peers, as this can undermine their self-esteem and confidence. Celebrate their strengths and accomplishments and encourage them to focus on their progress.

- **Neglect self-care:** Parenting a child with ADHD can be stressful and demanding, so it's essential to prioritize self-care. Make time for activities that recharge your batteries, such as exercise, hobbies, and spending time with supportive friends and family members.

- **Hesitate to seek support:** Don't hesitate to seek help and support when you need it. Whether it's from a therapist, support group, or other parents of children with ADHD, connecting with those who understand your experiences can be invaluable.

By implementing these do's and don'ts, you can create a supportive and nurturing environment for your child, helping them thrive and reach their full potential. Remember to be patient, flexible, and compassionate as you navigate the challenges of parenting a child with ADHD.

Taking a Holistic Approach

Taking a holistic approach to managing ADHD involves recognizing that proper nutrition is just one part of the puzzle. For a thorough approach to your child's well-being, it's crucial to integrate nutritional interventions with other tailored strategies to meet the varied needs of children with ADHD.

- **Therapy and counseling:** Therapy provides crucial support for children with ADHD, aiding in coping strategies, self-esteem, and emotional management. CBT, play therapy, or family therapy can all be beneficial.

- **Educational support:** Educational support, like IEPs, ensures children with ADHD receive the necessary accommodations for academic success. Collaborate with teachers and counselors to create a plan addressing your child's learning style and challenges.

- **Behavioral interventions:** Behavioral interventions teach ADHD-affected children skills to manage behavior, improve self-regulation, and develop social skills. Options include behavior modification, social skills training, and parent programs.

- **Sleep:** Ensure your child gets consistent and sufficient sleep each night. Sleep is vital for your child's physical and mental health.

9–11 hours of rest per night can improve attention, impulse control, and mood regulation, helping to mitigate ADHD symptoms and promote overall well-being.

- **Exercise:** Encourage your child to engage in regular physical activity, such as outdoor play, sports, or active games, for at least 60 minutes per day. Physical exercise supports cognitive function, reduces hyperactivity, and enhances mood, improving ADHD management and overall health.

- **Mindfulness and meditation:** Introduce mindfulness practices or guided meditation sessions into your child's daily routine. These techniques can help improve attention, decrease impulsivity, and manage stress by fostering self-awareness and emotional regulation. Just 10-15 minutes of either practice daily can significantly benefit ADHD symptoms and overall well-being.

- **Creating a comprehensive plan:** You can make a holistic plan for managing your child's ADHD by integrating nutrition with therapy, education, behavior interventions, and lifestyle changes. Collaboration with healthcare professionals and educators is essential to customizing interventions for your child's needs.

Recognize that each child with ADHD is unique, and responses to nutritional interventions may vary. Stay patient and open-minded as you experiment with different dietary approaches, observing how your child's body and behavior react.

Prepare for challenges during implementation, such as resistance to new foods or inconsistency with dietary changes, and understand that setbacks are normal. View them as opportunities for growth and learning, persisting with patience and resilience to achieve long-term success in managing your child's nutrition and well-being.

Address potential challenges by adjusting your strategies, involving your child in meal planning, simplifying meal preparation, and preparing healthy options for social situations. Also, try to remain flexible with dietary strategies that will suit your child's needs and adjust them as necessary. Even small changes can significantly improve your child's health and well-being.

Finally, stay informed about the latest research and recommendations related to nutrition and ADHD. Seek reliable and evidence-based resources, engage in continuing education, collaborate with health care professionals, and remain open to experimentation and adaptation. Embracing ongoing learning and staying informed about nutrition and ADHD is crucial for effectively supporting your child's journey. You can optimize your child's nutritional health and well-being by staying engaged and seeking reliable information.

A Message of Hope and Confidence

As we conclude, let's reflect on your journey exploring nutrition's role in managing ADHD. We've shared practical strategies and evidence-based insights to empower children with ADHD to improve their focus, self-regulation, and well-being.

By combining nutrition with therapy, education, behavior interventions, and lifestyle changes, parents like you can create a holistic plan for children's needs.

Looking ahead, let's approach the future with hope. With the right interventions, children with ADHD can thrive. Let's stay committed to learning, collaboration, and adaptation, ensuring every child has the support they need to succeed. So, in closing, let's move forward with optimism, knowing that with the proper support, our children with ADHD can lead fulfilling lives.

Jake's ADHD Journey: A Tale of Resilience, Growth, and Advocacy

Throughout the chapters of this book, Jake's journey with ADHD has been a testament to resilience, growth, and the power of understanding and embracing each child's unique neurodiversity. From his struggles in school to challenges in social situations, Jake has faced various obstacles associated with ADHD. However, through perseverance, support, and a commitment to self-discovery, he has learned to navigate his condition with courage and determination.

Jake's experiences have highlighted the multifaceted nature of ADHD and the importance of adopting a holistic approach to its management. From exploring the impact of nutrition and lifestyle factors on symptom management to discovering the value of supplements and alternative therapies, his journey has encompassed a wide range of strategies for optimizing his well-being.

Additionally, Jake's story has emphasized the significance of self-acceptance and advocacy in the journey with ADHD. Through self-reflection and growth, he has learned to embrace his strengths and challenges and advocate for himself and others with ADHD.

In this book, Jake's experience inspires and empowers individuals with ADHD and their families. It illustrates the transformative potential of understanding and embracing neurodiversity, fostering resilience, and thriving despite ADHD's challenges.

Thank you for reading this book. This labor of love was born from a mother's care and concern for my son. I understand that many parents, like myself, are nervous and skeptical about giving medications to their children. Whether you choose to use medications or not, dietary and behavioral changes can make a world of difference in ADHD kids and adults!

Your feedback means a lot to me and helps others discover the benefits of this book. Please leave a review! Thank you for your support!

-Maya

References

ADHD and diet. (n.d.). Tees Esk and Wear Valley NHS Foundation Trust. https://www.tewv.nhs.uk/about-your-care/conditions/adhd/diet/

Alice. (2022, September 19). *The ADHD symptoms that may cause food-related struggles.* The Mini ADHD Coach. https://www.theminiadhdcoach.com/living-with-adhd/adhd-food

Arnold, L. E., Lofthouse, N., & Hurt, E. (2012). Artificial food colors and attention-deficit/hyperactivity symptoms: Conclusions to dye for. *Neurotherapeutics, 9*(3), 599–609. https://doi.org/10.1007/s13311-012-0133-x

Beckerman, L. (2022, March 30). *Picky eaters with ADHD: A parent's guide to mealtime.* ADDitude. https://www.additudemag.com/picky-eaters-adhd-parents-guide/

The best supplements for ADHD. (n.d.). MyDynamics. https://www.mydynamics.co.za/story/the-best-supplements-for-adhd/

Bradley, S. (2022, July 13). *The best ADHD diet.* The Checkup. https://www.singlecare.com/blog/adhd-diet/

Campain, A. (n.d.). *Decoding sugar on the nutrition fact label*. Kendall Reagan Nutrition Center. https://www.chhs.colostate.edu/krnc/monthly-blog/decoding-sugar-on-the-nutrition-fact-label/

Capanna-Hodge, R. (2023, October 20). *ADHD treatments: A holistic approach to managing your child's symptoms*. Dr. Roseann. https://drroseann.com/adhd-treatments-for-children/

Carpenter, J. (2022, October 12). *ADHD and diet: How nutrition can help ADHD symptoms*. D Amore Mental Health. https://damorementalhealth.com/adhd-and-diet/

Cickovski, T., Mathee, K., Aguirre, G., Tatke, G., Hermida, A., Narasimhan, G., & Stollstorff, M. (2023). Attention deficit hyperactivity disorder (ADHD) and the gut microbiome: An ecological perspective. *PloS One, 18*(8), e0273890. https://doi.org/10.1371/journal.pone.0273890

Daily exercise ideas for children with ADHD. (2016, November 28). A D D i t u d e . https://www.additudemag.com/slideshows/exercise-ideas-for-kids-with-adhd-movement-for-focus/#:~:text=Get%20children%20moving%20after%20school

Ede, G. (n.d.). *Food sensitivities and ADHD*. Diagnosis Diet. https://www.diagnosisdiet.com/full-article/food-sensitivities-and-adhd

Fernando, N. (2022, November 21). *How to tame your child's sweet tooth: Tips for parents*. Healthy Children. https://www.healthychildren.org/English/healthy-living/nutrition/Pages/How-to-Tame-Your-Childs-Sweet-Tooth.aspx

Flannery, S. (2023, March 6). *What we know about ADHD and food*. Child Mind Institute. https://childmind.org/article/what-we-know-about-adhd-and-food/

Friendships: Teenagers with attention deficit hyperactivity disorder (ADHD). (2022, September 15). Raising Children Network. https://raisingchildren.net.au/teens/development/adhd/friends-friendships-teenagers-adhd

Gill, K. (2023, June 1). *ADHD diet for kids: Which foods can help and which to avoid*. Medical News Today. https://www.medicalnewstoday.com/articles/adhd-diet-for-kids#which-diet-is-best

Government of South Australia. (2012). *What can I do as a teacher or school to encourage healthy eating habits and to be active?* https://www.sahealth.sa.gov.au/wps/wcm/connect/public+content/sa+health+internet/healthy+living/healthy+communities/schools/what+can+i+do+as+a+teacher+or+school+to+encourage+healthy+eating+habits+and+to+be+active

Grabmeier, J. (2022, May 19). *Diet plays key role in ADHD symptoms in children*. Ohio State News. https://news.osu.edu/diet-plays-key-role-in-adhd-symptoms-in-children/

Hjalmarsdottir, F. (2020, January 30). *Does nutrition play a role in ADHD?* Healthline. https://www.healthline.com/nutrition/nutrition-and-adhd

How to manage ADHD: Lifestyle factors that improve symptoms in children. (n.d.). ADDitude. https://www.additudemag.com/how-to-manage-adhd-without-medication-kids-lifestyle-poll/

Iliodromiti, Z., Triantafyllou, A.-R., Tsaousi, M., Pouliakis, A., Petropoulou, C., Sokou, R., Volaki, P., Boutsikou, T., & Iacovidou, N. (2023). Gut microbiome and neurodevelopmental disorders: A link yet to be disclosed. *Microorganisms, 11*(2), 487. https://doi.org/10.3390/microorganisms11020487

Kahn, A. (2023, May 18). *5 tips to help kids with ADHD handle peer pressure*. Understood. https://www.understood.org/en/articles/adhd-tips-peer-pressure

Kids, C. (2023, November 4). *ADHD and gut health*. Catch Up Kids. https://www.catchupkids.co.za/adhd-and-gut-health/#:~:text=In%20individuals%20with%20ADHD%2C%20there

Lange, K. W., Lange, K., Nakamura, Y., & Reißmann, A. (2023). Nutrition in the management of ADHD: A review of recent research. *Current Nutrition Reports, 12*(3), 383–394. https://doi.org/10.1007/s13668-023-00487-8

Mayo Clinic. (2017). *What nutrients does your child need now?* https://www.mayoclinic.org/healthy-lifestyle/childrens-health/in-depth/nutrition-for-kids/art-20049335

Meal planning for the child with ADHD. (2016, February 4). Parenting Hub. https://parentinghub.co.za/advice-column/parenting/meal-planning-for-the-child-with-adhd/

Myers, W. (2023, December 5). *5 foods to avoid if your child has ADHD*. Everyday Health. https://www.everydayhealth.com/adhd-pictures/how-food-can-affect-your-childs-adhd-symptoms.aspx#:~:text=Many%20parents%20wonder%20if%20artificial

Newmark, S. (2012, November 28). *Eggs, dairy, nuts, and soy: Testing for food sensitivities with an ADHD elimination diet*. ADDitude. https://www.additudemag.com/testing-for-food-sensitivities-in-children-with-adhd/

Newmark, S. (2019, December 3). *The best ADHD diet for kids & adults: Healthy foods for ADD*. ADDitude. https://www.additudemag.com/adhd-diet-for-kids-food-fix/

Orenstein, B. W. (2023, October 17). *Best healthy snacks for your kid's ADHD-friendly diet and worst foods to avoid*. Everyday Health. https://www.everydayhealth.com/adhd-pictures/healthy-snacks-for-kids-with-adhd.aspx

Pearson, K. (2017). *How Omega-3 fish oil affects your brain and mental health*. Healthline. https://www.healthline.com/nutrition/omega-3-fish-oil-for-brain-health

Pinto, S., Correia-de-Sá, T., Sampaio-Maia, B., Vasconcelos, C., Moreira, P., & Ferreira-Gomes, J. (2022). Eating patterns and dietary interventions in ADHD: A narrative review. *Nutrients, 14*(20), 4332. https://doi.org/10.3390/nu14204332

Porter, E. (2017, October 13). *Parenting tips for ADHD: Do's and don'ts*. Healthline. https://www.healthline.com/health/adhd/parenting-tips

Roybal, B. (2008, May 13). *ADHD diet and nutrition*. WebMD. https://www.webmd.com/add-adhd/adhd-diets

Rucklidge, J. J. (2018, September 28). *Do diet and nutrition affect ADHD? Facts and clinical considerations*. Psychiatric Times. https://www.psychiatrictimes.com/view/do-diet-and-nutrition-affect-adhd-facts-and-clinical-considerations

Saline, S. (2021, July 15). *Dinnertime for the family with ADHD: How to make family meals more enjoyable for all*. Dr. Sharon Saline. https://drsharonsaline.com/2021/07/15/dinnertime-for-the-family-with-adhd-how-to-make-family-meals-more-enjoyable-for-all/

Schaefer, A., & Yasin, K. (2020, April 29). *Is sugar an addictive drug?* Healthline. https://www.healthline.com/health/food-nutrition/experts-is-sugar-addictive-drug#What-is-an-addiction?

Sonderegger, A. (2023, September 29). *How to treat ADHD without meds*. Neuro Wellness Spa. https://neurowellnessspa.com/how-to-treat-adhd-without-meds/

Tacoma, N. (2019, March 11). *Mindfulness and ADHD: 4 relaxation games for children*. ImpactParents. https://impactparents.com/blog/adhd/mindfulness-and-adhd-4-relaxation-games-for-children/

Watson, S. (2008, May 27). *ADHD and substance abuse*. WebMD. https://www.webmd.com/add-adhd/adhd-and-substance-abuse-is-there-a-link

Wirth, J. (2023, June 6). *ADHD statistics*. Forbes Health. https://www.forbes.com/health/mind/adhd-statistics/#:~:text=The%20average%20age%20for%20an